# *Relax* your **Neck**
# **Liberate** your *Shoulders*

## The Ultimate Exercise Program for Tension Relief

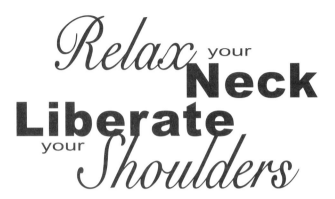

# Relax your Neck Liberate your Shoulders

## The Ultimate Exercise Program for Tension Relief

Eric Franklin

Elysian Editions
Princeton Book Company, Publishers

# For my parents, Joan and Jules Franklin

Please note: this book can help you become more flexible, provides information, and can help you help yourself. It does not replace medical advice. If in doubt, or experiencing acute pain or suffering from illness, consult a doctor or other qualified health practitioner.

Originally published as *Entspannte Schultern, gelöster Nacken*
©2000 für die deutsche Ausgabe by Kösel–Verlag GmbH & Co., München

Elysian Editions
Princeton Book Company, Publishers
P.O. Box 831
Hightstown, NJ 08520-0831

Translated by Francis Shem Barnett and Arja Laubaucher
Photographs by Eric Franklin
Illustrations by Sonja Burger

Cover, layout design and composition by Lisa Denham

Library of Congress Cataloging–in–Publication Data
Franklin, Eric N.
    [Entspannte Schultern, gelöster Nacken. English]
    Relax your neck liberate your shoulders: the ultimate exercise program for
tension relief. / Eric Franklin.
       p. cm.
    ISBN 0-87127-248-2
    1. Neck pain—Exercise therapy.  2. Neck pain—Prevention.  3. Shoulder pain—Prevention.
4. Shoulder pain—Exercise therapy.  5. Relaxation.  6. Massage. I. Title.
RD763 .F7313  2002
617.5'3062—dc21
                                 2002035601

Printed in Canada        8, 7, 6

# Contents

# Acknowledgements

For the inspiration for my work I would especially like to thank Mira Alfassa, Sri Aurobindo, the teachers of ideokinesis, and especially André Bernard. I would also like to acknowledge Bonnie Cohen, The School for Body Mind Centering®, its wonderful teachers and, and last, but not least, all my students and teachers at the Institute for Franklin Method. My thanks go to the illustrator Sonja Burger for her excellent realization of my drafts, the unknown back silhouettes of New York, the elastic fellow beings who agreed to model for photos, and the translators Francis Shem Barnett and Arja Laubacher who did a fabulous job of converting difficult German phrases into eloquent English. My special thanks to Princeton Book Company, Publishers, for the realization of the project.

# Preface:
# Keeping the Noodles on the Fork

**A** while ago I flew from Zurich to San Francisco. People sat quietly in their seats, reading their newspapers. One man exclaimed that there was smoke coming out of the wings: condensation trails. The flight attendant tried to calm him down. Everyone was eating and watching a movie: an angel fell in love with Meg Ryan and he jumped off a skyscraper to become human so he could feel her kisses. She was frustrated because he didn't feel anything; as an angel one is freed of all physical sensations. One cannot feel pain, but likewise nothing beautiful—that was the story line.

The physical exercise on the plane consisted of going to the toilet, waiting outside the toilet, and maybe a little stretching to look out of the window to see how the condensation trails were doing. I wondered to myself how I could expect to arrive in San Francisco feeling like a human being if that was all the exercise I was going to get. I certainly didn't want to land as an angel. I'd rather be a human being who feels his joints creaking, with a stiff back and tense shoulders.

I don't exaggerate when I say that before the flight my head was balancing on a completely loose neck. It actually felt as if it was free of gravity and it was a pleasure to turn my head since my neck felt so supple, my shoulders were as light as fluffed feathers, and my breathing was free and deep. What I would have liked to do most was dance. Instead I had to go through a ravine–like entry gate into a silver cylinder. I was surprised at how intensely pleasant my body felt as I boarded.

Even though it's my job to help people to feel good in their bodies, I am not always in this exquisite state, which I had no intention of losing on a twelve–hour plane journey. I came prepared: I had my ability to visualize, I had two exercise balls, and last but not least a copy of the manuscript of this book—stored in my memory.

Of course there were amused looks when I did my exercises on board. But it seemed more important that my muscles were being amused than that I was perceived as a normal passenger. Every time I felt even the slightest tension arise (for example one had to press one's arms up against one's body in order to be able to eat without nudging one's neighbor's noodles off his fork), I did an exercise.

All the tension in my body literally flew away over the clouds. I was the master of my physical state, and this had a very positive mental effect. The flight didn't annoy me with its seemingly never–ending length. There was always something to do. I felt comfortable.

After the flight, despite twelve hours on the plane, I enjoyed the way my body felt.

# Introduction

## Ideokinesis: Exercising with Internal Imagery

The philosophy of this book is based on ideokinesis, not to be confused with kinesiology. Applied kinesiology, or "Touch for Health," is a method that is based on reflex points and muscle feedback. In ideokinesis, using imagery for the development of body awareness is primary.

Ideokinesis goes back to Mabel Todd and her pioneering book, *The Thinking Body* (first printed, 1937, latest edition, 1997). At the start of the twentieth century, Mable Todd had an accident that paralyzed her. The doctors had given her up as a hopeless case, but she didn't give up and continued to exercise with what was left to her: her imagination.

Mabel Todd healed herself, and learned to walk again — with even better coordination than before her accident. Although, in those days, it was so unusual to work with imagery, she made use of this huge area of potential for posture and movement improvement. Soon students and patients were flocking to her, and she healed many so–called hopeless cases.

Now ideokinesis is taught at many universities in the USA, and is standard practice for many gymnasts, as well for teachers of dance and kinetics. It is also applied by physiotherapists, and is used in normal day–to–day life. At my Institute I have further developed the art of ideokinesis and now call it the Franklin Method. I have added many exercises, images and movement as well as exercise balls and Thera-Bands® to the repertoire. Since many areas of the body were not fully explored in original ideokinesis, such as the pelvic floor, knees, and feet, I have added information on these areas. This book also draws from other excellent modalities such as Body Mind Centering® (BMC)[1], the Zvi Gotheiner Teaching Method[2] and concepts from Integral Yoga[3].

---

1 Body Mind Centering®, founded by Bonnie Cohen in 1973, teaches movement through anatomical, physiological, and developmental principles.
2 Zvi Gotheiner, choreographer and dance educator in New York, has developed his unique method of teaching ballet based on sensory awareness, correct alignment, and movement efficiency.
3 Integral Yoga, developed by Sri Aurobindo in Pondicherry, India, encompasses body, mind, and life: "All life is Yoga."

The Franklin Method is about better coordinating the hidden strengths of the body and creating the basis for efficient and gentle movement. Its aim is to not only improve what we have, but to improve what we can become through changing structures, so that we can feel and move more harmoniously right down to single cells.

Behind every unhealthy physical movement pattern slumbers a good one. But instead of getting tense by trying to change the bad, we delve into the body to bring the good back to the surface. Imagery serves as an echo sounder that encourages the body to rediscover dormant natural movement patterns. In this sense nobody is truly clumsy or cramped; poor functioning is merely a temporary dominance of inefficient coordination; in the background there is a better movement pattern waiting to be resurrected.

It's like the stage at a theater: we can see the backdrop of a forest on the stage, but behind it there is a castle waiting to be used in the next scene. Even though the castle (better coordination) never disappears, we can only see the forest (deficient coordination). We try to change the forest into a castle, but this is much too difficult; it is a lot easier to simply discover the castle behind.

Our path is a very intuitive process, and is not based on a particular map. Human beings are much too complex and individual for a route to be dictated by someone else. For every person, a different set of rules applies. This is not a problem, however, because the body is always willing to reveal its "plan of the day."

The main purpose of this book is to kickstart the dialogue with the body via various experiments and exercises. That way, tension is no longer the enemy, but a message from the body and a potential for learning.

Later in these pages I will describe just such a dialogue with the body.

Teaching imagery exercises is like a balm for the whole body, because one is relaxed, coordinated and centered while teaching. The exercises are passed on through the teacher's own subjective experience, and an automatic self–correction system develops in the student.

When the time is right, the body sends whatever messages are needed to our awareness in the form of images and perceptions. Our surroundings become an inspiration: the cells of the body orientate themselves on an image of fluttering leaves, or a bubbling brook inspires us to be more flowing and relaxed. While exercising with imagery, we experience how mental states are connected with the perception of the different bodily systems. The experiences we have of our muscles, for example, create a different mental state than the experience of the organs, joints or nervous system.

The harmonization of the various physical systems gives our thoughts more flexibility, and images and insights about our mental patterns can surface more intuitively. Instead of demanding of the body healthy behavior, or prescribing exercises like pills, there occurs a dialogue with the body as between equals. Physical problems such as persistent back tension, headaches and arthritis, are dealt with at their root, and we can find our own individual, personal solutions. We can make swift progress in our training as we uncover and eliminate unfavorable movement patterns.

For this to happen, the will to take responsibility for oneself is needed, as well as curiosity, imagination, and taking a great interest in exploring the body. It is important to remember that the body can heal itself, it just needs the right encouragement. The appropriate "topic of the day" is usually decided by the body, and is always full of surprises. In the next section I will talk about such images and ideas that came upon me on two different days.

Let's start on the next page with an example of a spontaneous imagery experience.

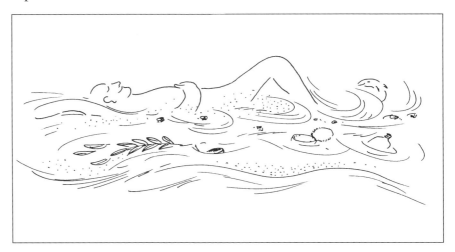

## magical self–correction

It's a bit like a fairy tale. One day I was walking along a street and all of a sudden I felt a widening at the back of my pelvis. It just happened by itself, I didn't do anything. The small of my back widened, the tailbone (coccyx) lengthened, and a wonderful feeling of looseness spread throughout my lower back.

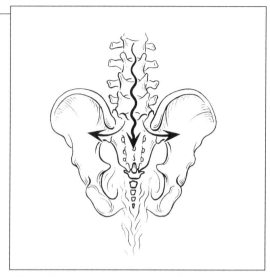

I could feel how the bones at the front of my pelvis were gently pushed together, which in turn took the weight off my back. My legs swung in perfect alignment back and forth as I walked. I could feel clearly how the heads of my thighbones lay deep in their sockets. And most surprising of all, both my ankle joints relaxed at the same time, and my feet became completely loose. Taking each step was a wonderful feeling, and I could have continued walking like that forever.

I continued to walk in a circle, even though I had arrived at my destination. I thought: "I don't care if other people are watching me, I want this feeling to get anchored deeply in my nervous system, so that it will become a permanent movement pattern."

## thinking patterns

That's how I spontaneously discovered truly relaxed walking, a free and upright posture, relaxed shoulders, and deep breathing. The experience showed that this new movement pattern was anchored deep in my being. Up until that moment all my exercises were only outer correction, and the tension already there was reproduced by my behavior again and again.

### undisturbed sand

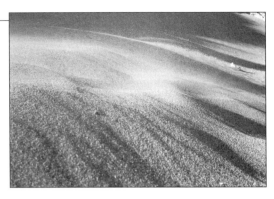

Sit down comfortably on a chair and imagine that your body is very calm and untouched, like a big stretch of sand. Every thought can potentially disturb the sand like a strong wind—a furrow is created, sand dunes heap up, and the smooth surface is all stirred up.

Start with a few trial thoughts. Imagine something very pleasant, an agreeable situation, and see if this disturbs your stretch of sand. Now imagine an unpleasant situation and again observe the effect this has on your stretch of sand. Is it possible for the surface to stay undisturbed? Now let your thoughts roam freely. Keep your inner eye on the sand and watch whether it is possible for the sand to stay undisturbed. You can have thoughts, but they do not stir up the sand.

## structure of this book

This is both an exercise book and a reference guide. You may choose a new relaxation technique each day or read it through from cover to cover, trying out all the exercises in the order presented. Naturally you will want to repeat the exercises that work best for you, but I recommend integrating them, occasionally, with new ones.

There is a method for everyone. Exercises with or without visualization, exercises with different levels of difficulty, exercises with or without props, and exercises with both an anatomical and a psychological/spiritual orientation. Some exercises teach you to use imagery, thus awakening more body awareness. These are for your experimentation. I invite you to start with the exercise series for beginners and then experiment.

*These exercises are not presented in terms of a right way or a wrong way.* Your thoughts and feelings influence the effectiveness of the exercises you do. If you are afraid of doing something wrong, you are, of course, going to be tense right away. You will broaden your movement potential by approaching the exercises with curiosity and without demanding immediate perfection. If an exercise feels uncomfortable, it doesn't mean that it was executed incorrectly—it may simply be that you are not yet ready for it. Just move on to the next one. Experiment!

*Where does tension come from?*

Almost every exercise in this book addresses a particular cause of neck and shoulder pain, whether it is biomechanical, emotional, or a combination of the two, *with the emphasis on practical relief.*

*An image for the neck and shoulders*

When I ask my beginning students for positive images of their shoulders and necks, their answers are often "no pain," or "relaxed." Relief of tension is so much more complex than merely an *absence of pain*. We find that we have oriented our bodies to the words *no pain, no tension* and *no inflexibility*. Unfortunately this focus is on pain, tension and inflexibility! This book will guide you to positive and appealing visions and images.

Here are some examples of causes of tension and pain and corresponding constructive visions:

| Cause of tension and pain | Positive image |
| --- | --- |
| narrow thinking | A sense of well–being in the neck and shoulders frees my thinking. |
| not enough movement | My muscles are working harmoniously and every movement is a joy. |
| bad posture and coordination | Centered strength inhabits my body, my joints are free, my physical system is stable. |
| stress, not enough time | I am calmly mastering my daily life. |
| no interest in my body | My body and mind feel supple and flexible. |
| exhaustion, sluggishness | I have energy and a lust for life. |
| no joy in my job | Every job is a joy. |
| discontentment with my general situation | I can feel growing contentment in my soul. |
| no trust, lack of intuition | I have spontaneous and intuitive thoughts which show me the way. |
| headaches, migraines | My head is free and light. |
| tensed breathing | My breathing is deep and relaxed. |
| unhappy with my looks | My looks are fresh and healthy. |

constant hyperactivity

I have a balanced metabolism and enough tissue breathing for detoxification.

Everyone has a specific mix of reasons for neck and shoulder tension. Therefore, this book offers a wide variety of helpful tools which will guide you to success. You will learn that the most important tools are responsibility for yourself and the development of body awareness, leading to perception—an early–warning system which helps you to detect and then correct problems before they become insurmountable.

## imaginary waterfall

Imagine you are standing underneath a waterfall. The water flows over your neck, shoulders, and back. All tension is washed away.

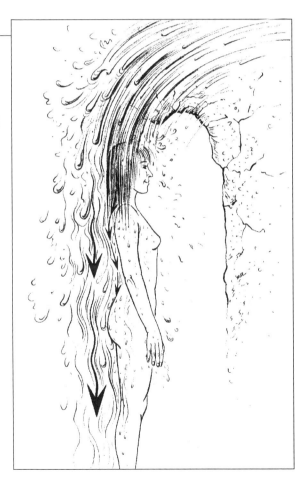

# 1  Tension

## tension as misinterpreted movement

One could say that tension is a place in the body that feels tight or hard, that hurts, or is knotted or cramped. Unfortunately this description does not help us much while trying to remove tension. Here's a better explanation: tension is a misinterpretation of movement. Where there should have been movement there was none and the result is tension. It comes about when our physical system has been geared to movement but none is made.

Here's an example: sometimes we get rebuked without cause. Our natural response would be to jump up and protest: "No, no, it's not true, that's not how it was! "But often this sort of reaction is not possible—perhaps we are sitting in the classroom as a child, or as an adult in front of our boss. The body is preparing to react, the muscles vibrate, waiting for release, but nothing happens; we continue writing in the classroom or leave our boss's office. Of course these are reactions, but physiologically insufficient ones.

One can argue that it is hardly realistic to start jumping up and down screaming at our teacher or giving our boss a few slaps. These reactions might well have consequences that could in turn lead to even greater tension.

### there are some possible solutions, however

**1.**  One can wait until later and then allow the appropriate reaction, for example hitting a pillow. Better late than never.

**2.**  One can learn to not tense up in reaction to unpleasant situations: one stays physiologically calm, even though one is being blamed unfairly. One way to do this is to concentrate on the center of the body, just below the navel.

**3.** One can become familiar with the responses of one's body, with which muscles and joints tense up in these situations. The more harmonious these muscles and joints are, the less one is charged with unnecessary anticipation.

## better late then never

Sometimes it is wiser to postpone one's reaction to a situation. So instead of becoming angry with the boss, we can go outside and jump up and down for a minute, shouting, perhaps. While doing this, don't think of the boss, but of how all the tension is flowing out of the body. Ideally there'll be no colleagues watching you! If there is no place nearby outside, you can also sneak into the photocopy room and tear some used paper to shreds. In this way one has supplied one's muscles with blood, instead of creating negative thought patterns about one's boss. For children it might be helpful in situations like this to beat up a cushion or have a tussle with dad.

## protection from tension

Tension has the annoying habit of returning again and again. One reason for this is that aside from recreating it inside ourselves, we also pick it up from our environment. One is especially vulnerable to absorbing other people's tension when we're tired or stressed out. One of my own experiences illustrates this nicely:

I was feeling very good one day. I was feeling happy and every joint and fiber in my body was feeling wonderful. My wife has a friend who works on a farm who came visiting that day with an injured leg. A horse had caused it when it was getting vaccinated. The upper part of her shin was broken and her knee was hurting. As I was able to visualize it very well, a certain unease came upon me—what if this had happened to me? That same evening my own knee started to hurt.

Over the weekend I was able to cure it, but then later I treated my son who had a problem on the ball of his foot. The next day my foot hurt, though my son's was fine. Although I felt tired and uncentered I managed to heal my foot.

Three days later I had dance rehearsals. A dancer came in with a stiff neck and that same afternoon so did I.

Were these merely coincidences? By then I could only laugh at it. I felt as if I was a pain–absorbing sponge.

**how do you stay relaxed when everybody around you is tense? there are two ways:**

**1.** Avoid people who are tense, and don't feel guilty about it.

**2.** Make sure your own relaxation is deep enough so that nothing in your environment disturbs it. Your relaxation is anchored both in the body and the mind.

The following exercises and ideas can help to protect one's own sphere of relaxation, even when surrounded by a lot of tension.

### staying relaxed in the jungle of tension

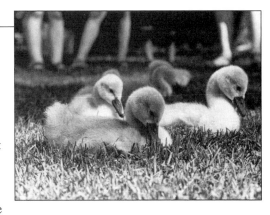

This partner exercise can be done with a bit of humor. Stand opposite your partner and move together with a lot of flow and suppleness. It is helpful to play some appropriate music. Then start moving with a lot of tension but continue looking at each other — the music should be turned off or changed to some tense music, like hard rock or techno. Then try to do the opposite of what your partner does: one makes soft loose movements, the other makes tense movements. Each tries to stay with his/her mode of movement. The goal is to get the other person to fall out of his/her movement mode. Then reverse roles: the one who moved flowingly now has to move with tension, whereas the one who was tense now moves softly.

Afterwards shake your body thoroughly – arms, legs, trunk and head.

Through this exercise our ability to stay relaxed in a tense environment is greatly enhanced. Next time you meet a tense person just think to yourself: "It's astonishing how easy it can be to stay relaxed in unfavorable circumstances with this technique, and even to experience how flowing life can be."

One morning I had the feeling that the whole world around me was somehow softer than usual. The buildings and the cars were soft, the streets and the trees, everything seemed softer and more supple. Actually, from an objective perspective it was not a particularly nice morning: it was drizzling, the streets were wet, it was dark and cold.

Of course, I was aware that according to normal perception I had hard stone under my feet and the buildings around me were not made of rubber at all—but still, everything seemed to be soft and elastic that morning. I enjoyed this perception thoroughly. The whole happening felt utterly regenerating and reminded me of the soft down of ducklings, who also surround themselves with softness.

Suddenly I noticed how everything seemed to proceed more easily. Even though there was a traffic jam it seemed as if I didn't have to wait, and the cars spread themselves out like pudding. When I had to make a turn, a space seemed to open magically. The ground under my feet was elastic, my step was springy, and the people I met seemed to be more easygoing than usual—physically as well as mentally. I felt that life was soft, flexible, elastic.

It occurred to me that conventional wisdom considers life to be "hard." Of course, if you see it like that then it will most likely be like that. But I had experienced something else that day, and I said to myself: "It wasn't an intellectual decision that I made to perceive things like that; it simply happened to me."

### surround yourself with softness

In this experiment focus your awareness on the space around you. Imagine that the air is very soft, it is flowing cosily around your shoulders; it feels as if it was a silk scarf. Say to yourself, "I am breathing this soft, pleasant, light air. I have my own sphere of lightness. I will try to carry this soft coat around me the whole day; when something hard comes towards me, I will stay soft and won't absorb any of the hard stuff."

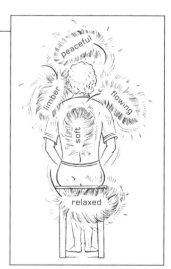

## time pressures and time robbers

When one has the feeling that there isn't enough time to do what one thinks one has to do, then one is under time pressure. This is a familiar situation for many people.

One day when I had to finish a lot of things I started thinking about the phrase, "time pressure." I felt the physical effect of time pressure like a compression in my body cells, a tension in the area of the heart and the shoulders. Since I had had some experiences with the softness of life, I asked myself if there was an opposite phrase to time pressure.

I didn't find one, so I tried to invent one: time enjoyment, time abundance, gift of time, time joy, time excess, time delight, time relaxation... Something became clear to me right away: in everyday usage all terms to do with time have negative connotation. These considerations alone were enough to lessen the feeling of pressure I was experiencing. Just listing the potentially positive aspects of time had brought that about.

Two days later I attended a conference with a colleague. She wanted to order a cappuccino in the break, but there was a big crowd around the beverage counter. The serving lady said, "I can't make any cappuccinos now, they take too long." I thought, "Aha! Time theft!" Who has not experienced this before? To make a cappuccino would take time that would be better divided up into small slices to prepare three teas or coffees, instead of just one cappuccino. The belief that something has to be done quickly, because otherwise one is doing less, or loses time, leads to the biggest loss: time abundance (or is it "the joy of time?").

## time abundance

Breathe in and out deeply and remember that time is endless: a never-ending source of time is magically bubbling up. This source is at our disposal at all times; time spreads out in front of us like an eternal golden carpet. The more we are able to bathe in that feeling, the better our cells will feel.

# 2  Relaxation for Beginners

In the following section we will start exercising with movement, breathing and imagination. We can profit best from the following exercises if we focus on the body during them. An important factor is "centering," an inner concentration that enables us to feel the body as a whole and to coordinate our movements. In the following experiment we will start with becoming aware of the energy around our body.

## a ball of energy in the hand

Rub your hands together until some heat develops. Then hold them about 2 cm (an inch) apart and focus on the space between the hands. Start with breathing into and out of this space, and then imagine that you are passing an energy current from one palm to the other.

After one or two minutes move your hands slowly towards each other, and then away again. It may be that you can feel a pressure, warmth or suction between your hands, that the space between the hands feels magnetic, or like a ball of energy. (If you are not sure whether you can feel something, move one hand upwards so that the palms are no longer facing each other. You should notice the magnetic field by its absence.)

With the magnetic field between your hands you can give your body something good, give it an energy present. If there is a place in your body that is tense or needs energy, place your hands there. You can also touch two places at once. Imagine that these places are recharged with energy and relax. Another possibility is to cross your arms and put your hands on the shoulders and feel how the energy of your hands relaxes the shoulders in this protected space. It's best not to do this while wearing a thick sweater because the arms get pushed away from the body.

## organs create flexibility

In the following experiment we shall see that the relaxation and energetic charging of an organ has a direct bearing on our flexibility. We will be using visualization, touch, and our voice. The kidneys are a key organ for the relaxedness of the whole body and should be taken care of daily with the use of awareness.

### energy for the kidneys

As described before, rub your hands together until warmth is produced. Move the palms away from each other 2 cm (an inch) and feel the energy there. After a minute put the left hand on the kidneys on your back (near the bottom rib).

Put your right hand underneath the same rib on the front of the body. Visualize a stream of energy flowing through the kidney from one hand to the other. Thus you offer the nourishing energy of your hands to the kidneys. Guide your breathing to the kidneys so that they feel carried and supported. Visualize the fact that the kidneys are a filter that takes all the waste out of our blood, and we want to support them in this task. Our blood is refreshed like water from a spring that is filtered and purified by moving through many different layers of stone.

We can awaken our kidneys by singing a deep Aaaahh. Imagine that they start to vibrate with this sound. After about a minute let your arms swing loosely by your side and feel the difference between the two halves of your body. Is the left shoulder more relaxed? Does the left foot feel like it has a better stance?

Lift the left knee, and then the right one. Which leg is easier to lift? Hold your arms straight up in the air. Which shoulder feels more relaxed? And finally, turn your upper body to the left, and then to the right — which side is it easier to turn to?

In a variation of this exercise we put both hands on the kidneys at the back. Breathe into the kidneys and imagine that they become wider and relax to the rhythm of your breathing. As you breathe in, think of your back billowing like a sail.

After a few minutes take the hands away and feel how the back and shoulders have relaxed.

## the balance between being and doing

When we finally have the time to actually feel ourselves, it is as if our sensory system has fallen asleep and we have to stimulate and wake it up by training it. If we can support it throughout the day, we will have better concentration and more energy. For this, the important thing is not the quantity but the quality of the perception.

## being instead of doing for one minute

Stand in a relaxed position and focus on your feet. Feel the feet relaxed on the floor. At the same time give free rein to your breathing, don't hinder it in any way. Observe which parts of the body your breathing moves: chest, belly, back, pelvis, arms, legs. Watch your inner eye as it moves around your body.

Focus on the growing inner peace and try not to interfere intellectually. It is as if we are soothing a child by becoming calm ourselves. Simply observe the body—every cell in your body and brain is relaxed.

Now let everything go, including the inner observation.

You just are, without doing.

# regeneration–a full–time job

We often think we have to do something in order to heal or improve ourselves. In reality our body is busy healing itself every moment; millions of immunity cells are constantly buzzing around purifying us inside. The pituitary gland, along with other glands and hormones, takes care of maintaining a perfect homeostasis. If this stopped for even a short time we would not survive. Trillions of cells are constantly busy creating new protein.

In just the time it takes to read these lines, thousands of cells are born by cell division. Every organ is recreating itself all the time. You are a completely new human being from the one you were some years ago: almost every cell of your body has been replaced. The main activity of the body is rejuvenation and regeneration.

You can trust completely in this process.

## renewal

Rather than focusing on ailments, try to live the following idea: "My body is healing itself every moment. All the cells of my body are constantly refreshed and refuelled. My body becomes more and more the embodiment of renewal and regeneration. I can trust it completely."

# relaxing the shoulders

Those muscles that are used to lift parts of the body are tense with most people. Because we carry our shoulders too high up, they suffer from chronic shortening. Two of these muscles are called the trapezius and the levator scapulae (see pages 41 and 47).

By carrying the shoulders too high, the spine gets overloaded, which makes the body unstable. And this all costs energy.

But if we relax the trapezius and the levator scapulae, our inner peace will grow, our breathing will become deeper, and we will be more grounded. We discover that inner calmness, letting things happen, and relaxation, are closely connected to our shoulders. Letting things happen doesn't mean just allowing everything, but rather dealing with daily life without tension. Life starts to flow, things happen by themselves, and we begin to attract helpfulness.

Surprisingly, it is helpful to focus on the shortening of the muscles before loosening and relaxing them. It's like getting away from the shore with a little boat: you have to push hard to get away from the shore.

In the following experiment we will be using our voice. It is an important ingredient of the exercise and its effects should not to be underestimated. In human evolution it was not the development of the hands or the brain that accompanied the change from quadruped to biped, but the changing of our vocal apparatus — the larynx, and the throat. An erect posture is a vital condition for language. Voice and language help us to stand up straight and remain erect.

### sighing shoulders

Lift your shoulders upward towards your head. Now lower the shoulders again very slowly. Feel how the muscle fibers are stretching like chewing gum. It is helpful to exhale when lowering the shoulders and to visualize the shoulder blades gliding down the back.

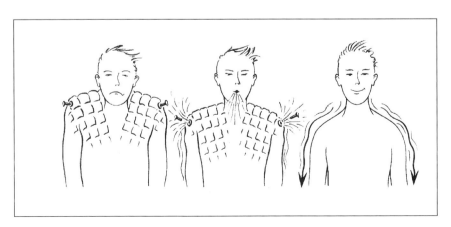

Lift the shoulders once more and feel the shortening and tensing of the muscles. Now leave the shoulders to gravity and allow them to be drawn down slowly—try to let gravity do the work. The muscles flow apart, head and shoulders separate. It almost feels like the shoulders could fall down to the pelvis.

Repeat the exercise again and at the same time sigh with a loud Aaah or Oooh while the shoulders sink down. It is as if the muscles are sighing as they say good–bye to all the tension, letting out all the air like emptying an air mattress.

Again, lift your shoulders and let them down. Picture all your problems falling to the ground, where they will be absorbed, recycled and will pop up again as wonderful flowers!

One last time, lift your shoulders and inhale, and let them down with a deep sigh. Let everything that you don't need fall to the ground—plump! Let your sorrows ooze away into the ground. Feel your head become free.

Open your body, make it receptive to the new and the good. Breathe in harmony and hope. Feel the elasticity of your chest and make an Eeeee sound—this sound helps to give the spine more length. Now feel the elasticity of your chest and make an Ooooo sound, which helps to give depth to the body. Feel the elasticity of your chest and make an Aaaaw sound—this helps to give to the body a feeling of lateral expansion.

## shoulders draping pelvis

Physically speaking, the weight of the shoulders lies, via the chest and spine, on the pelvis. In order to be able to feel this, imagine when lowering the shoulders that they are falling down to the pelvis. It is important to visualize the process and not just the final position. Feel the gradual lowering as a gentle process which keeps going, never stopping.

It is possible that, even though you think these shoulder exercises are great, you cannot make such liberal use of your voice without getting some tongues seriously wagging. And this could endanger your newly

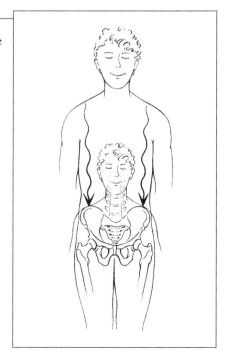

gained relaxedness. This is where the "drinking straw" experiment can be helpful.

## the drinking straw experiment (adapted from Carola Speads)

This exercise is very calming, has a relaxing effect on the nervous system, and deepens the breath.

Take a normal drinking straw and breathe out through it. Breathe in normally through the nose, while holding the straw in your hands—take care not to take deep breaths, as this can make you dizzy. The straw should not be held between the teeth, since this tenses the jaw and cancels out the positive effects of the exercise.

## shoulders and drinking straws

After doing the straw breathing for a while, you can go on to lifting the shoulders when inhaling and lowering them slowly when exhaling. Take care that the hand and arm holding the straw stays relaxed. Breathe in and out three or four times. Then take a break and look at how your shoulders, breathing, and body posture are. If done properly, this exercise is a veritable stress terminator. If you don't have a straw handy, just let the shoulders down with a slight hissing sound. It is important to breathe normally, i.e. not too deeply, and to not continue with the hissing for too long.

## tapping

Tapping with the hands is a very simple and effective technique. It enhances the circulation, and detoxifies and relaxes the muscles.

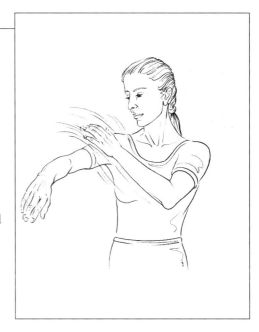

To tap, hold the fingers slightly extended, allowing the wrist to be as elastic as possible; the wrist should stay relaxed with each tap. When doing this exercise, be totally concentrated on the area that you are touching.

We start the tapping exercise with the belly. After tapping around the navel clockwise, move your hands in the direction of the digestive tract, following the rising colon on the right side of the body upwards. Tap on the horizontal colon from right to left side at the height of the upper belly. Tap on the left side of the body, following the descending colon downwards and across the lower belly from left to the right. Repeat this circular tapping movement about three times.

Now tap on all sides of the right arm. Start with the palm of the hand and tap upward to the armpit. Continue to tap on top of the shoulders descending to the hand. From there tap from the thumb on the inner edge of the arm right up to the collarbone. Now only the outer edge of the arm is left: tap from the shoulder blade outwards to the little finger. Before doing the same on the other arm, compare how both arms feel. Does the left arm feel lighter and more relaxed? How are your shoulders?

Now repeat the exercise on the left arm.

This exercise can of course also be done with a partner.

Next, tap on the head. Be careful and keep your finger joints very loose. Feel the skull bones vibrating lightly under your fingers.

During the tapping, give special attention to the cheekbones and to the jaw, which should hang loosely—also relax the tongue.

Now softly tap the breastbone, which activates the thymus gland. When activating the thymus gland it is helpful to make an 'Aaahh' sound while exhaling. This organ is an important agent of our immune system. The tapping and sounding widens the upper chest and makes an erect posture feel effortless.

Without a partner the upper back is not easy to reach. When tapping the lower back, exhale with a loud Ooooo and form the hands into loose fists.

The legs should only be tapped where one can comfortably reach. Tap the front of the legs from the hip to the toes. Return to the pelvis by tapping on the inside of the leg from the big toe to the pubic bone. From the side of the pelvis, tap on the outside of the leg down to the small toe. Touch the heels and tap on the back of the legs, moving upwards. Imagine how the cellular fluid in the muscles vibrates with your tapping movements. To focus on the liquid element in our muscles is an important healing agent.

## arm shaking

Muscles are not rigidly fixed to the bones. They are able to move around the bones to an astonishing degree. They are packed in layers into connective tissue bags. These bags relay the contractile action of the muscle to the tendons and bones. It is due to their ability to shift within these connective tissue envelopments that our muscles remain mobile.

When we shake our arm, it helps to restore the flexibility of connective tissue and muscle and improves the distribution of the body fluid.

Tension is not only found in muscles and connective tissue; blood and lymph vessels, ligaments, bones and tissue can all become tense. Through the following exercise, tissue becomes lubricated and thus internal body space management is improved. To put it differently, relaxation can spread, like distributing sand evenly on a plate by lightly shaking the plate.

When we shake the arm, the ligaments, tendons, vessels, bones and bone marrow are all moved, as well as the muscles. Even the nerves are moved. Awareness of movement disperses tension.

### shaking arms, shaking legs

Hold the right arm out in front of you, parallel to the ground. Shake the arm and imagine the muscles swinging around the bones, fluttering loosely like the sleeves of a large shirt. If you want, you can also visualize other tissue being shaken: vessels, bone marrow, red and white blood cells.

I like to concentrate on the delicate nerve endings. I imagine that they get shaken and dusted like a feather duster that is shaken out of a window. The nerve endings free themselves of tired old feelings, so they are free once more for new things.

Before shaking the left arm, compare the feeling in both sides of the body. Often there are astonishing differences—it's amazing what a good shake can do!

One can do the same exercise with the legs, just with the added difficulty of balancing while standing on one leg. I recommend doing the exercise while sitting down, holding the edge of a chair with both hands while shaking the leg.

Feel free to experiment with different speeds and intensities of shaking— from a fast shaking or vibration to a movement like the light kicking of a ball.

Can both legs be shaken with equal ease?

# 70% water

The human body is 70% water. Most of this water is found in the body cells, which can be visualized as tiny water reservoirs. The rest consists of inter-cellular fluid, blood, lymph, and cerebrospinal fluid (the liquid around the brain and spinal cord). The human body produces an astonishing amount of its water itself, in the mitochondria of the cells. The mitochondria are the power generators of the cells. A "byproduct" of power production is water. The shoulders are three-quarters water—but how can water get tense?

## rippling in the shoulders

Try to visualize all the water that is in our body: trillions of tiny water reservoirs in the form of cells, and several miles of blood vessels. All this liquid produces streams, eddies, whirls, rapids and quiet pools.

Now move your body and focus your attention on all the liquid in it. Feel how this liquid murmurs and ripples in your shoulders; as you move your shoulders, you are sending many small waves through trillions of cell pools. Feel how blood permeates all the capillaries in the shoulders. Every tissue is steeped in liquid.

A further image to picture is that of the harmoniously arranged rice fields in the Chinese highlands—thousands of little pools in a terraced arrangement.

# discrimination and discernment

The following exercise is about discrimination and discernment. We will learn to differentiate between the different parts of the body that are involved in the movement of the arms and shoulder girdle. The more "discrimination" we have of the body, the more flexible we are. If all we can discriminate and feel of our body is one big lump, then we will hardly be flexible.

We often do exercises to become more flexible in those areas that are already the most flexible. To become looser throughout our body, it makes more sense to develop the "stuck" places by visualizing them and starting our movements from there.

Each part of the body is represented in the brain. Through actually moving those parts of the body that are tense, this representation becomes reintegrated into the control mechanism of the nervous system. Then we can be consciously flexible in those areas. In this exercise we will be engaging the organs, which have a crucial influence on our flexibility.

### locomotivation

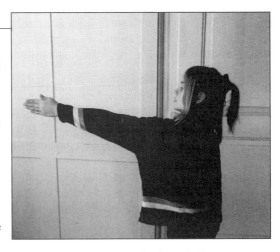

This exercise can be done either standing up or sitting down.

Imagine that the arms, shoulders and lungs are like a locomotive pushing a train from behind.

Start with the right arm. Hold the hand up just in front of your chest. Push the hand outward, using the lower arm. Then push the arm even further out using the upper arm. Now push the whole arm further outwards with the shoulder blade. And now the finale: imagine that the soft filling of the thorax, lungs, and heart push the hand outwards even further. While doing this, imagine the content of the thorax is honey, and that the hand is grabbing a beautiful peach hanging in the air.

Now let the arms swing a bit, stretch both arms out side by side, and compare their length.

## shaking the diaphragm

The diaphragm is a dome with a boomerang–shaped aponeurosis (flat sheath of connective tissue) as a roof and a ring–shaped wall of muscles. It is attached to the spine, the breastbone and the ribs. The right side of the diaphragm lies slightly upwards due to the proximity of the biggest organ, the liver.

Similar to the arm–shaking exercise above, in this exercise we will swing the diaphragm to relax it and so it is better supplied with blood. It is more difficult to shake the center of the body than a limb. For belly dancers this is not difficult, but for the rest of us it is something of a challenge. But we will gladly take up this challenge, since by loosening the diaphragm the shoulders relax and spontaneous laughing emerges.

### the diaphragm swings

Rapidly rotate the thorax and the shoulders back and forth around your axis This is a quick, swinglike movement and it should be accompanied with an Aaaah sound. If this sound becomes rhythmic through the rotational wing, we have been successful with our exercise.

Jump gently up and down and make sure that you bend the knees to cushion the landing. Imagine that the diaphragm is a trampoline stretching up and down, reacting to your movement. Breathe out slowly: Aaaah. This breathing should become rhythmic through the movement of the diaphragm. Imagine that the shoulders sink down to the diaphragm, and during this sinking, the diaphragm floats like an autumn leaf falling off a tree.

## stretching the diaphragm

The diaphragm is perhaps the most important muscle of our body. Without it we would probably not survive for more than three minutes. So I have often wondered why this muscle tends not get any conscious stretching, as for example do the thigh or the calf muscles.

In the following exercise we will make up for this and we shall incorporate this muscle into the illustrious "stretching club."

Visualize the fibers of the diaphragm in the thorax: they lie in an almost vertical direction underneath the ribs

The area where the diaphragm and the ribs are opposite each other is called the opposition zone. Since the fibers of the diaphragm shorten when we inhale, this zone then becomes smaller. When breathing out, the fibers of the diaphragm stretch and so the zone gets bigger. To stretch the diaphragm, we concentrate on the lengthening of the muscle fibers on the inside of the ribs.

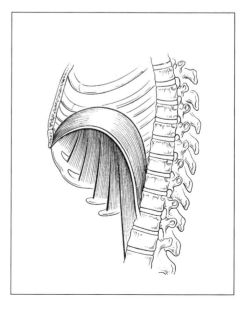

### stretching the diaphragm and the lungs

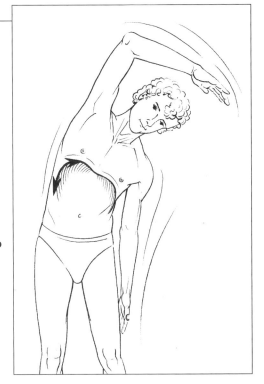

Hold your right arm straight up and put your left hand on the right side of the thorax. Visualize the diaphragm under your hand and bend the upper body to the left when exhaling. Both feet should be anchored solidly to the ground. Imagine how the fibers of the diaphragm are stretching. When inhaling, stand straight again.

Repeat: when exhaling, bend to the left; and when inhaling move back to the upright position. Repeat this bending/exhaling and straightening/inhaling four or five times.

After doing this exercise, one often notices astonishing differences between the two sides of the body—more space in the lung, more relaxed shoulders, and even a looser jaw on the stretched side.

If we bend the upper body to the left and then to the right, we can feel that one side is much more stretched than the other, likewise turning the trunk to the left feels more elastic than turning the other way. You may also notice that the right arm feels longer now. If we stretch our arms up and imagine we are holding a dumbbell, it will be much easier for our right side because the relaxed diaphragm gives us more strength there.

Now repeat the exercise on the other side.

## collarbone massage

The collarbone is an S–shaped bone that connects the breastbone and the shoulder blades. Around the collarbone there are a lot of vessels and muscles. If we loosen up this area, it has a very beneficial effect on our breathing and our shoulders.

### liberating the collarbone

Lift your right shoulder a little, so that you can easily feel the collarbone with your fingers. Try to massage the whole bone, from the breastbone out to the shoulder blade. Move the shoulders in a circle and feel the movement of the collarbone. Try to loosen the muscles behind and under, too—do this carefully, as there are many points that are sensitive.

Afterwards, compare both sides and notice that a loose collarbone helps to relax the shoulders.

Repeat on the other side.

## the swing of the pendulum

This exercise is about learning to distinguish between the primary and secondary skeleton. The primary skeleton consists of the spine, skull and thorax. Evolutionarily, this is the older part of the skeleton, which also makes up the main part of a fish's body.

The secondary skeleton consists of the limbs, including the pelvis and shoulder blades.

There will be too much tension in the secondary skeleton if it is too tightly bound to the primary skeleton.

The goal is to reach a certain independence, and with it a constructive dialogue, between the two skeletal parts. In the following experiment we want to let the peripheral, or secondary, skeleton hang from our central, or primary skeleton. This way we can stay centered in our dealings with the outside world. People often look as if they are trying to achieve the opposite: to hold themselves up by the shoulders, neck and jaw, while the spine, thorax and pelvis are sagging. We concentrate on the activity of the outside (arms and legs) too much compared to the experience of the center (spine and pelvis).

### the arm hangs from the thorax (adapted from André Bernard)

Stand up and concentrate on your left arm. The arm hangs from the breastbone. To feel this more clearly, let the fingers on the right hand walk up the left arm, starting at the left hand. Say to yourself while "walking" up the arm and shoulder: "The hand hangs from the lower arm; the lower arm hangs from the upper arm; the upper arm hangs from the shoulder blade; and the shoulder blade hangs from the breastbone." Try to feel the weight of the different parts of the arm and to let them hang from each other like parts of a mobile.

Imagine that the arm is a thick rope and bend the upper body to the left. Visualize how this rope is hanging from the breastbone, and start to swing the arm back and forth from the breastbone. The feeling is of a long pendulum that is attached to the breastbone. Try to move the pendulum as effortlessly as possible.

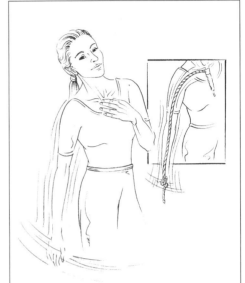

Put your hand on the collarbone and feel how it is moving back and forth with the arm. Swing your arm for about two minutes until you have the feeling that the arm is really swinging from the breastbone.

Now comes an important moment: straighten up again from the breastbone while the arm stays hanging. Don't lift from the shoulder, but from the center of the breastbone. Compare both shoulders and repeat the exercise on the other side.

After the exercise, the arm hangs consciously from the joints and bones, so the muscles can relax completely. This can create a permanent lengthening of the shoulder muscles. (For more information on this topic, see my book *Dynamic Alignment through Imagery.*)

## swinging from the floor

Stand with your legs spread as wide as the hips, with knees slightly bent. Try to swing your hands back and forth from the wrist joints. Allow the swing to rise up your arm, so that now the lower arm is swinging from the elbow. Finally, swing the whole arm from the shoulder. Now try to anchor the swinging even deeper in the body: swing the arms from the collarbone and breastbone, and then from the spine.

Trigger the movement from the pelvis and pelvic floor, from the legs and finally from the feet and the ground. Now your swing is grounded and your arms integrated right to your feet. After the exercise, while standing quietly, try to experience how your arms are supported by the ground. If you can find this feeling, it unburdens the shoulder and spine muscles to a great extent. The resulting grounding reminds us also of the goals in T'ai Chi and other Far Eastern movement arts.

# feet and shoulders

Livening up the feet does wonders for the shoulders. It is highly recommended that you use every opportunity to loosen and strengthen the feet. The more active the feet are, the more the shoulders can thrust and release. In a way, it is as if the shoulders cannot relax because of the lack of strength of our foundation, as if they are trying to compensate by tensing up. If a house has a bad foundation, the walls and the roof suffer because of it. The same is true of the human body: the feet, the pelvis and the spine are the substructure of the shoulder girdle and the head. This foundation needs to be in harmony if the shoulders are to be relaxed and free of tension.

When the shoulders' condition is improved, the lower levels begin to remedy their defects. The body always functions holistically—it is only our intellect that separates it into different functions.

The following exercise can be done inside your home or outdoors.

### standing on a towel or root

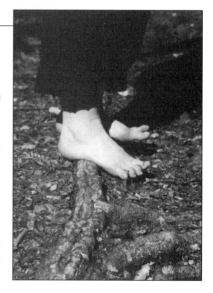

Take a medium–sized towel and wind it into a compact roll. Place this roll on the floor and stand on it with both feet. If you feel unstable, you can lean a little against a wall. You may also use a pair of small balls that I have designed for this and many other exercises called the Franklin Ball.

Breathe freely and move your legs and feet around a bit, bend your knees and wiggle your toes.

For nature lovers, try standing on a tree root. I recommend taking off your shoes and starting with a smooth root. As above, keep moving, breathe freely and keep the toes relaxed. With practice you'll be able to stretch your whole body, to lift your arms, and even to close your eyes.

### balancing on a towel or root

Whenever we move in a way that challenges our sense of balance, our nervous system is intensely exercised. The reflexes that constitute the basis of our coordination are honed and learn to support our movements efficiently. If we can stretch and challenge our sense of balance simultaneously, the result is astonishing, and the effect of the stretching is greatly increased.

Standing on your rolled towel, root, or Franklin Balls (see page 108), stretch sideways as described in the diaphragm–stretching exercising (page 17). As you're standing on unstable ground, holding your posture will be somewhat tricky. Nevertheless, try to relax and breathe freely (though when doing the exercise for the first time this will not be easy!) After about half a minute, go back to your starting position on steady ground.

Compare both shoulders and stretch your arms in front of you, above your head.

You'll probably notice that the stretched side is more relaxed and is able to breathe more deeply. When bending to the other side, you'll see how inflexible it is in comparison.

# friend tension

Let's assume that you did all the above experiments and exercises and still feel some persistent tension. Firstly, I recommend that you continue with the book, doing further exercises and regularly repeating the exercises you know.

But there is something else you can do.

Try to see this tension, this knot, this pain, as a friend and not as an enemy—a friend who has come to draw your attention to something; a friend who will not go away just because you are in a bad mood, one that takes the time to help you uncover the root of the problem. In doing this a dialogue will begin in which you not only ask questions, but also answer them. In the following experiment we will assume that the tension is in the shoulders, but this concept can be applied to any part of the body.

## hi, muscle knot!

Say the following: "Hi, Muscle–knot! You're still there. How strong you must be to stay tense for so long so that my nerves can feel this pain. Why are you so tense?"

# 3 Refresh your Joints

**O**ur body is more complex than any machine, but many of us understand it less than our car. Every musician knows all the intricacies of his instrument—without a well–tuned violin of good quality the violinist's talent would not be able to shine.

The following is a "manual" for the shoulders.

In four–legged animals the shoulder girdle rests on the "forelegs." For the adult human the situation is reversed: the shoulder girdle is the suspension for the "forelegs," or arms, and provides a stable base for our arm movements. This base, including the arms, only constitutes 10 % of the weight of our body. The joints and muscles of human beings and animals are similar but are used quite differently.

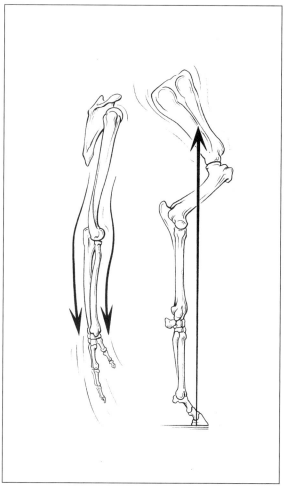

In the realm of joints, we find the main anatomical difference between humans and animals in the hands. The hand is only able to act as it does because of a dynamic shoulder girdle.

Two contrary aspects need to be combined: firstly, very fine coordination (for example when we write), and secondly, plenty of strength and stability (in order to be able to lift a baby stroller into a car). Astonishingly, the shoulder girdle, along with its attached arms, is connected to the torso by a relatively small joint. This increases our flexibility greatly, but also means that the stability of the shoulder girdle is chiefly the responsibility of the muscles. It is characteristic of the body that where it needs much flexibility, it achieves this primarily via its musculature. And exactly here lies the problem: how to move the muscles, which play such an important role in stabilization, in a relaxed and loose way? The answer is to recognize how the shoulder girdle fulfils its complex tasks, by experiencing it with awareness in daily life, and by trying to improve its function at every opportunity.

Let's start with the bones and the joints.

## the nature of joints

The point at which two bones meet is called a joint. This point is surrounded by a joint capsule and many ligaments. The ligaments and the form of the joint decide how flexible the joint will be. The ends of bones are covered with cartilage—a pressure–proof and lubricating material. Between the two cartilage surfaces there is what is called "synovial fluid." The cartilage and the synovia provide an almost friction–free area in the joint.

When our joints feel stiff, it is usually not due to the state of our joints but to our cramped muscles.

When the joints do actually become inflexible this is due to a pathological change in the cartilage surfaces—for example rheumatism or arthritis. Since cartilage does not have its own blood supply, it is nourished by the synovial fluid and through the underlying bony surface; but there is only enough nourishment if the joint is moved every day and regularly.

### flexibility of the shoulders

Wave your right arm in the air and focus on your shoulder. Now make a fist and feel what changes occur in the shoulder. Move the arm and the fist together. Now relax your hand and feel how the shoulder is more flexible.

The body functions holistically, so we are only as flexible as the least flexible part of our body. Our movement is always a general coordination throughout the body.

### flexibility of the hips and tense shoulders

Stand in a relaxed manner and bend your hip joint by lifting your knee as far as is comfortable. Make a note of the height of the knee. Put the leg down again and feel your hip joint. Now lift both shoulders and tense the shoulder muscles. Once more, lift the knee up. Now make note of how high you can lift the knee under these circumstances.

Tension in the shoulders makes us less flexible in the hip joints. If our hips are tense, we compensate in the lower back, which can lead to pain in the lumbar region.

## the shoulder girdle

The shoulder girdle consists of four bones: two shoulder blades and two collarbones. The collarbone is a delicate, S–shaped bone. One could say it is a shock absorber between shoulder blades and breastbone, and connects our arms to the side of our body. The collarbone of a cat or dog is short, and the arms do not swing from the side of the body but constitute the forelegs. Thanks to our long collarbones, which make sure the arms stay on the side of the body, the movement of the arms does not disturb the thorax. Likewise, our arm is more flexible because of the length of the collarbone, compared to an arm connected directly to the breastbone. Some of the muscles connected to the collarbone are often not flexible enough: the big and small pectoral muscles, the sternomastoid muscle (see page 98) and also parts of the trapezius muscle (see page 44).

The shoulder complex consists of four joints: the connection between upper arm and shoulder blade; the connection between shoulder blade and collarbone; the connection to the thorax between collarbone and breastbone; and the connection between the shoulder blade and the thorax, which moves like a joint, but doesn't have synovia or a joint capsule.

### the book stays in the same place

Take a book in your right hand and hold it in front of you in the air. Now try to move as much as possible while the book stays in the same place — the upper body, the legs, the shoulders, the arms, the whole body should be moved while the book stays relatively still. Before trying this out with the other arm, check the difference between both shoulders and arms.

## the shoulder blade

Many people complain about tension in the upper back between the shoulder blades. Often it extends painfully up to the neck and into the shoulders. The reasons for this are manifold. Many of the neck muscles begin at the upper back, and the shoulder blades are connected to the cervical spine, the head, the thorax, and the neck by many muscles and ligaments.

The outline of the shoulder blade resembles the outline of Africa with a prominent mountain range crossing it from one coast (Atlantic Ocean) to the other (Red Sea). This mountain range is the spine of the scapula and was originally the upper edge of the shoulder blade but has now folded downward. At the end of the mountain range is a cliff that overhangs the head of the upper arm bone. This cliff is called the acromion.

The shoulder blade is situated at the height of the second to seventh ribs. The inner edge of the shoulder blade runs almost vertical and is about five centimeters from the spine. The outer edge runs diagonally outwards from the bottom tip, and at the top towards the shoulder joint. Inside, the shoulder blade has a spongy appearance caused by miniature interconnecting trusses of bone. This makes the bone light while increasing its stability. The lower tip of the scapula points to the tuberosities of the ischium, also called the sitz–bones from the German "sitzbeine."

There are sixteen muscles attached to the scapula and they all vie for its favor. In this respect it is only surpassed by the lower jaw which has twenty muscles attached to it. Mabel Todd recommended imagining a weight attached to the tip of the shoulder blade so that it is pulled downwards, thus acheiving a lengthening in the muscles right up to the neck.

The more muscles there are, the more potential there is for tension. The posture of most people's shoulder blades is in fact too high and too far forward. The shoulder blade is the anchor and the foundation of all arm movements: it helps us when lifting the arm, just like a counterweight. Without it we would have to heave the arm up with sheer muscle power and our neck would look like Arnold Schwarzenegger's!

Even though the shoulder blades lie mainly on the back of the thorax, they have several connections to the front of the body. The most important is the acromion, which bends elegantly towards the front of the body to the dizzy heights above the round head of the upper arm in order to connect itself to the collarbone. So, the shoulder blade has, in fact, only one joint–based connection with the rest of the body—and that is on its front. On one hand the shoulder blades hang on the back, on the other hand they are connected to the front via the collarbone. We should take advantage of this and let the shoulder blades rest on the collarbones, which also act as shock pads. The collarbones stop the shoulders from falling inwards, and the more we use these resilient spacers, the less we have to use our muscles to stabilize the shoulder blades while moving the arms.

## currents in the shoulder blade

Imagine that there are several currents flowing in the shoulder blades just like in the ocean. The shoulder blade is not an inanimate object, but alive with eddies, whirls and waves.

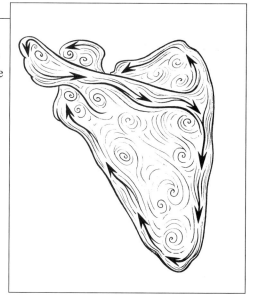

## shoulder blade, flapping of the wings

Hold your arms in front of the thorax at the height of the heart. Hook your fingers to create a firm grasp between your hands, elbows at the same height as the hands. Draw the elbows out to the side, but the hands stay holding each other. Now move the shoulder blades apart—the back bends forward when doing this. Draw the shoulder blades back again— the back stretches, the breastbone moves forwards. Imagine that the shoulder blades are wings that we are trying to flap up and down.

Repeat this movement five to ten times, making sure that you move as flowingly as possible and that you always breathe in a relaxed way.

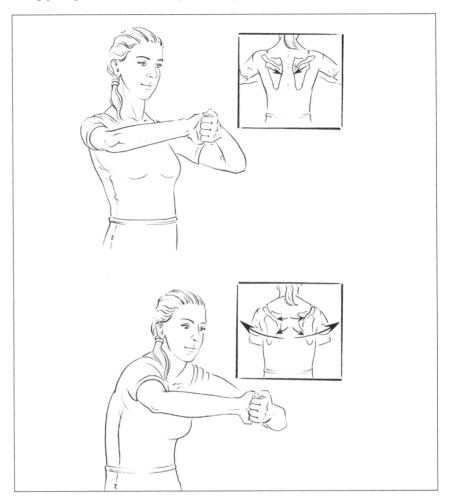

## lifting and lowering the shoulder blades

Interlace your fingers and face the palms away from the body. Stretch your arms to the front, making a slightly bent back. Now lift and lower the shoulder blades, paying special attention to the lowering. Feel the feet on the ground and breathe deeply. If you do not breathe calmly, you may become tense. Don't force the movement, even if you can only lift and lower the shoulders a little. Repeat the lifting and lowering five times, then let the arms swing loosely at the side of the body. Feel the effect of the exercise in the upper back and shoulders.

## circling shoulders

Put the back of your hands on the pelvic bones just below the waistline. To achieve this your elbows will bend at about a 90–degree angle. Press the hands lightly down onto the pelvis and make as big circling movements with the shoulders as possible. Imagine that your joints are well greased, and do the circling movement five times in each direction, forwards and backwards. Let the arms hang at the side of the body and focus on the release in your shoulders.

## shoulder blade and collarbone

Touch the joint. connecting the right shoulder blade and the right collarbone with your fingers.

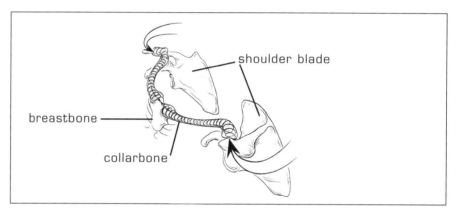

This connection can be found on the front side of the shoulder and feels like a small cleft. Bend to the left and move the right shoulder and arm up and down. Feel the movement in this joint, it contains a small wedge–shaped disk. Imagine how the shoulder blade rests on the collarbone. Feel how the collarbone pushes back on the shoulder blade.

Repeat the experiment on the other side.

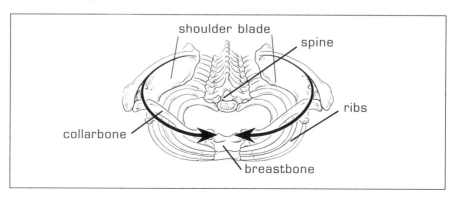

The collarbone is a sort of elastic block that lies like a shoetree between the breastbone and the shoulder blade and makes sure that the arms do not slip forward. Often, when having a bad posture, people try to pull the shoulder blades back and downwards—this is only making the situation worse! You need to change your alignment from inside out, through awareness and not by force which increases tension.

Instead, make circling movements with the shoulder blades forwards to the collarbone and to the breastbone, and feel the connection between the joints. It is similar to the pelvis, where the two halves of the pelvis come together in front of the body in the pubic symphysis. So, don't pull the shoulder blades back—on the contrary, feel how they rest on top of the breastbone via the collarbones.

### floating collarbones, falling shoulder blades

Imagine that your collarbones are being carried by balloons attached to the outer ends of the bones with fine threads. The arms hang, the collarbones float.

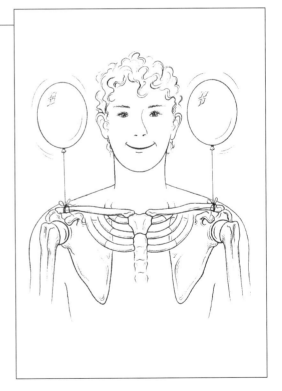

After being grounded for a while in the feeling just described, take a break from visualization, delete all images on the screen of your inner eye. Walk around and feel the posture of your upper body. And then, enjoying a bit more freedom in the upper body, imagine that the head and thorax are floating, light as balloons, arms and shoulder blades falling downwards.

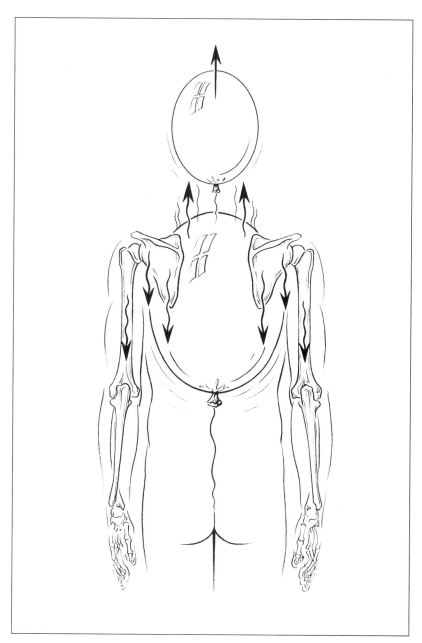

## movement of the shoulder blade

The shoulder blade can make many different movements. When moving, it slides on the thorax and is kept in place by many muscles. The shoulder blade can be lifted (elevation) and lowered (depression); it can glide outwards (abduction) and inwards (adduction). The shoulder blade can also be rotated in such a way that the joint socket faces upwards—the lower tip of the shoulder blade moves away from the spine and back again. This is an essential movement in lifting the arm.

Interestingly, the axis of rotation is shifted in the shoulder blade during rotation. It moves along the spine of the scapula outwards and up, almost to the acromion. This is why it feels like a pendulum swinging when lifting the arm. It also means that the shoulder blade sinks down when the arm is lifted. To feel that the lifting of the arm is a lowering of the shoulder blade is extremely valuable for reducing tension.

There are two other movements that the shoulder blade can make which can cause an imbalance in the muscles if they are too strongly developed. The first is a tipping backwards of the inner shoulder–blade edge ("making wings"). If this movement is developed too strongly, it might be due to a weakness of the rhomboid muscle (see page 50). Normally when lifting the arms in front of us the rotation of the shoulder blades is around a vertical axis. To enable this, the shoulder blade has to glide around the thorax, at the same time rotating towards the front of the body.

The second additional movement is similar to that of a raft on a wave. The thorax is like the top of a wave, since it is rounded. So while it glides upwards, the shoulder blade will sink into the valley of the wave, which is the upper ribs. During this, the lower tip of the shoulder blade is lifted. The reverse happens when lowering the shoulder blade: the tip sinks towards the thorax, the spine of the scapula moves backwards, and the shoulder blade stands almost vertical. Without this additional movement, the shoulder blade would move away from the thorax and be unstable.

The above movements are never made on their own but always in combination with some other movement—the lifting of the shoulder blade for example is usually connected with a slight rotation.

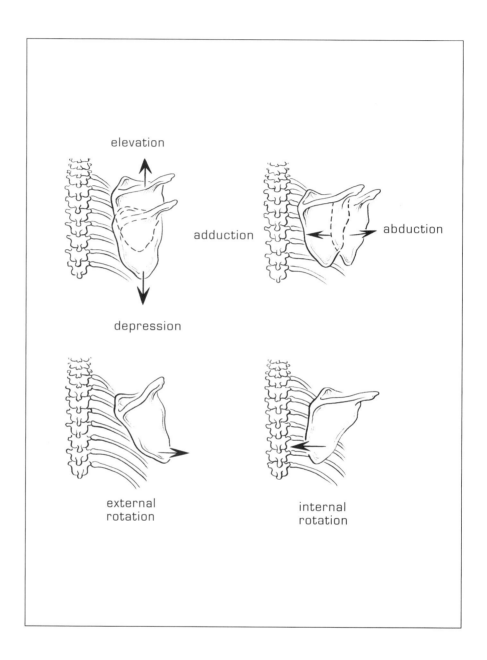

### swinging the shoulder blade

Touch the spine of the scapula at the point right behind the acromion. This is the axis of rotation of the shoulder blade when the arm is lifted. Lift your arm up and imagine that the shoulder blade is swinging like a bell, sinking a little while doing so. A partner can support this feeling by stroking the shoulder blade. When our imagination is powerful enough this will help relax the whole shoulder.

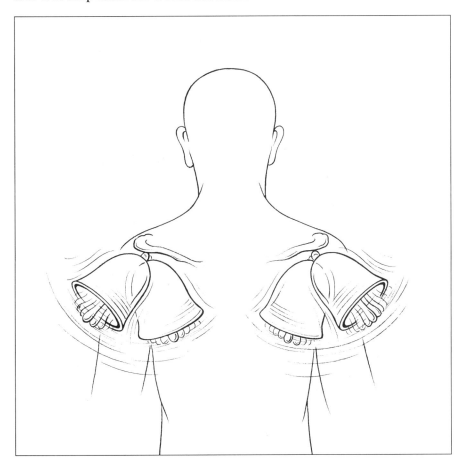

## humeroscapular rhythm (H–rhythm)

The humeroscapular rhythm is not a new Afro–Cuban melody, but a description of what happens when lifting an arm. It is a subtle combination of upper arm movement in the shoulder joint and rotation of the shoulder blade on the thorax. Without this rotation of the shoulder blade and the resulting upward facing of the shoulder socket, lifting of the arm more than 90–degrees would not be possible. The ball of the upper arm would impinge on the acromion. A similar situation can be experienced when trying to look at the ceiling by only lifting the eyes without turning the face upwards. The eyes can't see the ceiling unless the head moves as well.

Problems with this H–rhythm are the source of a lot of shoulder and neck tension. If the H–rhythm isn't working properly, we have to hold the entire shoulder girdle up, which adds considerably to the load of the neck and shoulder muscles. We can transform any exercise in which the arms are held up into loosening–up therapy if executed appropriately.

The H–rhythm has the following functions: an arm movement can be distributed between two joints; when the arms are raised, the ball of the upper arm can rest in a well–positioned socket and won't slip; and the muscles of the shoulder girdle do not have to take on extreme muscular elongation or shortening.

### partner exercise H–rhythm

Your partner puts his or her fingers on the lower tip and spine of the scapula. When lifting the arms, this tip moves outwards and the spine tips down and outwards.

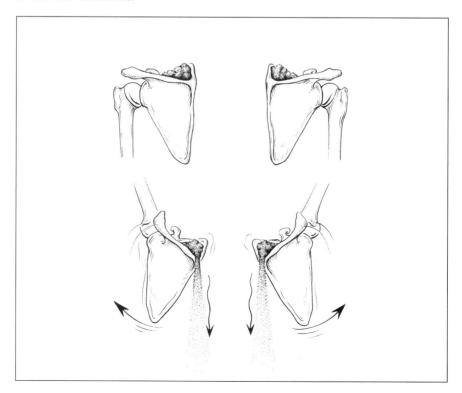

The shoulder blade forms a counterweight to the arm. This saves energy: instead of using lots of muscles to lift the arm, we let the shoulder blade drop as a counterweight. While doing this, imagine how the rhomboid muscle (see page 50) and the horizontal part of the trapezius are stretched.

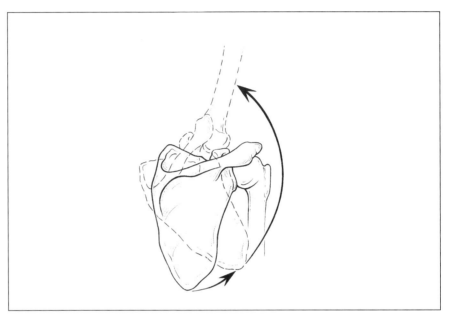

Support the movement of your partner's shoulder blade with your fingers by pressing the spine of the scapula down while he/she lifts the arm, and pressing the inner edge of the shoulder blade outwards with your thumb.

To feel what happens when the shoulder blade is blocked, do the following: firmly hold the shoulder blade by its lower tip. Now your partner is forced to shorten the shoulder musculature when lifting his/her arms. Afterwards, again help with the turning of the shoulder blade. It should now be much easier.

When the arm is stretched upwards, we can feel that it is sitting comfortably on the shoulder blade, like a building on a foundation.

And to finish with, an exercise done while standing up.

Put your hands on the shoulder blades of your partner. While he or she lifts the arms, stroke the whole back of the body right down to the heels with your hands. Both you and your partner should imagine that the shoulder blades are slipping down to the ground. You may imagine the shoulder blade to be a lathery piece of soap sliding down your back until it touches your heels.

### dumping sand

Imagine that there is a small heap of sand on the spine of the scapula. When lifting your arm this sand falls down along your spine. Hear and feel how the sand falls, taking with it all the tension.

## the coracoid process

There is a further connection between the shoulder blade and the front of the body. It is called the coracoid process.

This part of the shoulder blade, which looks like the rounded branch of a tree, peeps out from under the collarbone and lies next to the shoulder joint. Attached to it are three muscles: two lead to the arm, and the third—the pectoralis minor—is connected to the upper ribs. The shoulder blade lies like a knapsack on the back of the thorax, with straps that are attached to the front of the thorax. This arrangement has a lot of advantages, because the weight of the shoulder blade and arms is distributed evenly to the thorax. In theory this should make sure we've always got relaxed shoulders, but even this ingenious system is not able to overcome the stressed behavior of our species.

### shoulder blade as a knapsack

Touch the tip of the coracoid process by putting the thumb of the left hand into the dent under the collarbone and let it slide outwards in the direction of the shoulders. Inevitably we come against a hard, bony spot,

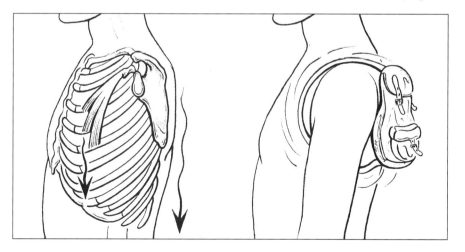

which we can feel with the ball of our thumb (the middle fingers of this hand should now be resting on the shoulder joint). This is the coracoid, which might feel quite sore, so do not press it too hard. Remind yourself that this spot is part of the shoulder blade. Thus something we associate with our back has a connection to the front of our body.

Now we stroke down and inwards diagonally to the upper ribs. This is the course of the pectoralis minor, acting like the strap of a knapsack (you might encounter some sore spots here). Imagine that the shoulder blade is carried via these straps to the front of the thorax. The shoulder blade is no longer fixed on the back, but attached to the front of the body.

Repeat the experiment with the other side of the body.

### sparkling eyes

Often the coracoid is pressed downwards due to a sagging upper body posture shortening the muscles that attach to it. Imagine now that the coracoid opens its "mouth" wide and yawns heartily in order to free itself from this pressure.

After this we imagine that the coracoid processes are small sparkling eyes, two cat's eyes glowing in the dark. These coracoid processes shine from under the collarbones, floating upwards and lifting the front a little, while the back hangs down relaxedly.

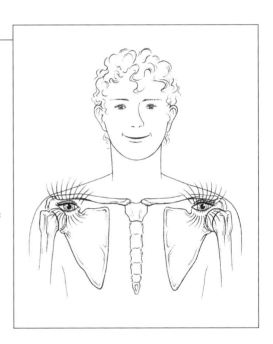

## finger to shoulder blade connections (after Bonnie Cohen)

To relax the shoulders and improve shoulder–hand coordination, it is very useful to be aware of the connection between the shoulder blade and the hand. This exercise helps to relax the shoulders and is a good preventative against carpal tunnel syndrome, as well as pains and inflammations that arise from monotonous work like typing.

### touching finger and shoulder blade

Start by clasping the thumb. Then stroke the fingers of the other hand along the inside of the arm up to the coracoid, which is the spot on the shoulder blade that corresponds to the thumb.

Now grasp the index finger and slide your fingers along the outside of the arm up to the spine of the scapula. This can be found on the back of the shoulder, on the top part of the shoulder blade — it is a long ridge that starts at shoulder level and continues towards the spine.

The middle finger actually corresponds to the socket of the shoulder blade. Grasp the middle finger and slide your fingers on the backside of your arm up to the acromion. Here, deep down, can be found the socket of the shoulder, which is part of the shoulder blade (glenoid cavity).

The fourth finger (ring finger) corresponds to the outer edge of the shoulder blade (margo lateralis). Slide your fingers from the ring finger along the outside of the arm up to the outer edge of the shoulder blade. Depending on the thickness of the muscles on top of it, it may or may not be easily felt.

The fifth finger corresponds to the lower tip of the shoulder blade (angulus inferior scapulae). First, grasp the little finger and slide with the fingers up along the arm and look for the lower tip of the shoulder blade. I recommend lifting the shoulder blade a little in order to find this spot. It is easier when a partner helps.

The wrist corresponds to the inner edge of the shoulder blade (margo medialis), the palm corresponds to the outward–facing plane of the shoulder blade, and the back of the hand corresponds to the inward–facing plane. Move all these areas of the hand and visualize the corresponding areas on the shoulder blade. If you want to relax the difficult–to–reach inward facing side of the shoulder blade, massage the palm.

I recommend again touching all the connections before making the comparison test: thumb: coracoid; index finger: spine of the scapula; middle finger: socket of the shoulder joint; fourth finger: outer edge of the shoulder blade; fifth finger: lower tip of the shoulder blade; wrist: inner edge of the shoulder blade; back of the hand: shoulder blade, outer plane; palm: shoulder blade, inner plane.

Now do the whole exercise on the other side of the body.

## the shoulder joint

Compared to the hip joint, the shoulder joint is very flexible. The task of the hip joint is to transfer the movement of the legs to the pelvis and to carry the upper body. Only when we are babies does the shoulder joint serve the function of a carrying joint; with adults it is mainly there to enable the three dimensional activity of the arms and hands. The stability of the shoulder joint is mainly due to muscles, unlike the hip joint, which uses a deep socket. But where a lot of muscles are used for stabilization, tension creeps in quickly. The shoulder joint is a ball and socket joint with freedom of movement in all directions. It is formed by the shoulder blade which provides the shallow socket (glenoid cavity) and the top of the upper arm bone, which provides the ball joint.

## movement in the shoulder joint

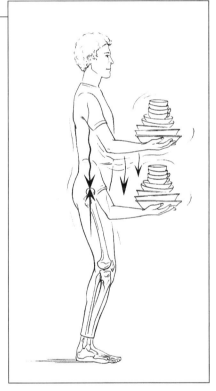

Feel an eye on the ball of the upper arm peeping into the shallow socket of the shoulder blade. This wonderful image was suggested to me by Glenna Batson, a physiotherapist and movement educator. All surrounding muscles provide a perfect centering of this bony head. It is a very slippery connection, and the shoulder blade can rest a little on the upper arm.

Lift the arm up sideways, and the ball rolls upwards in its socket. Soon it would push against the acromion. That's why the ball has to slide downwards for us to be able to lift the arm further. This is a so–called "gliding rotation." You can image the eye on the ball of the joint looking downward as you lift the arm.

If this gliding rotation didn't take place, we would have to move the whole shoulder girdle upward and bend sideways in order to lift the arm.

In our imagination we can exaggerate the gliding rotation a bit to accentuate it. Imagine that the ball of the upper arm slides down the side of the body until it comes to rest on the ball of the thighbone. It is no longer the shoulder girdle that is carrying the weight of the arms but the pelvis. Whenever we want to carry something with relaxed shoulders, this image is recommended.

# 4  Muscle Harmony

This book would not be complete without a discussion of the muscles of the shoulder girdle, an area we are often reminded of in a painful way. In the following exercises we will give them the attention they deserve and encounter them in a positive way.

The muscles of the shoulder girdle are arranged radially around the 'wheel hub' of the shoulder joint. This results in a lot of freedom in potential arm movements, but at the same time it takes a lot of effort and coordination for the spokes of the wheel to stay in balance. The shoulder muscles of the chimpanzee—our evolutionary ancestor—are built approximately the same way. Their job is hanging and swinging the body from branch to branch, whereas in our daily life the arms hang from the body. The shoulder muscles love to be used once in a while for their original purpose: to carry the body's weight.

This can be observed in children and in the great popularity of various types of climbing. To have a climbing installation in an office would be a great idea. This is why I will be presenting some exercises in the following chapter with exercise bands (see page 108) which make it possible to have this pull and push on the arms without climbing.

To move with ease does not require a lot of strength. The proverbial example is the baby. Its movements are very relaxed but it does not have a lot of strength. Strength is therefore not the key to relaxed movement, but nevertheless fitness training is often confuses it with strength training with weights. The basic conditions for lightness in movement for adults are body awareness, coordination, and the ability to imagine and picture one's own movement. If these elements are focused on while building muscle strength, then we can also move relaxedly with a lot of strength.

Mabel Todd, the founder of ideokinesis (see page xi), said that the architecture of the back muscles allows the shoulders to float.

Let's start with an image: the shoulder girdle is a mobile that is attached at the base of the head.

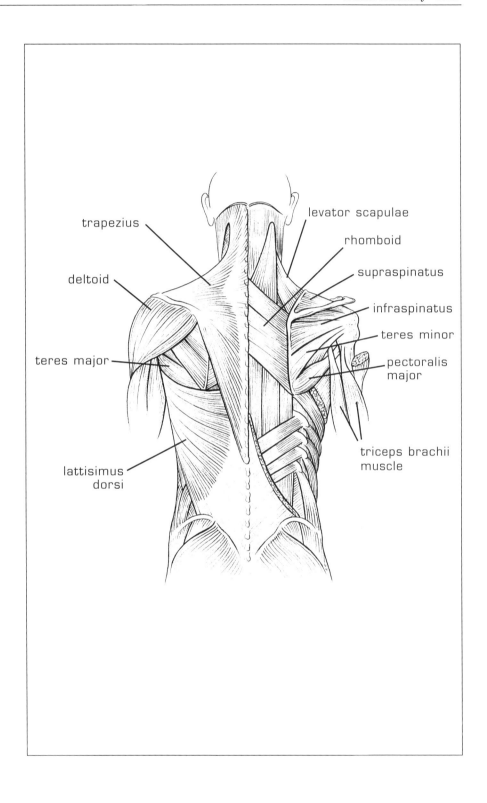

trapezius

levator scapulae

rhomboid

deltoid

supraspinatus

infraspinatus

teres minor

teres major

pectoralis major

triceps brachii muscle

lattisimus dorsi

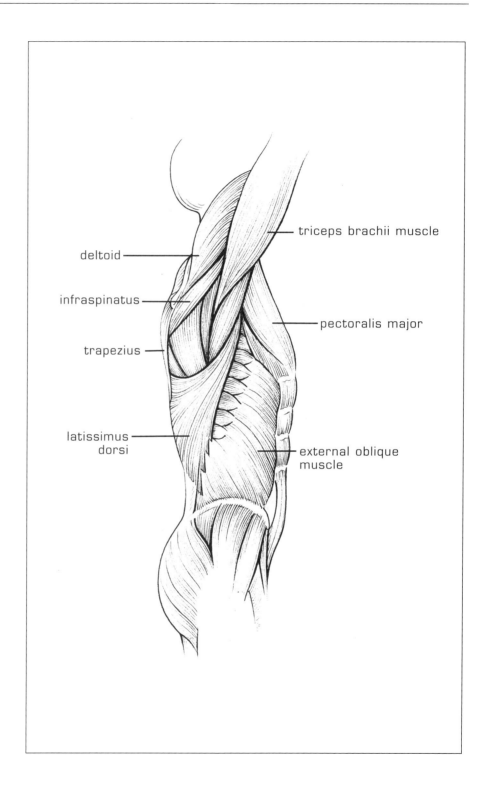

triceps brachii muscle

deltoid

infraspinatus

pectoralis major

trapezius

latissimus dorsi

external oblique muscle

# muscle sliding

To execute their complex movements the shoulder girdle and the arm are equipped with a lot of muscles. To improve the way they work we have to immerse ourselves in the language of muscles and get to know their basic functions. In this way we come closer to the nature of the musculature. In the words of Mabel Todd: "Structural Hygiene takes place when each structure finds its way back to its original function," and tension certainly doesn't belong with the original function of the shoulder girdle.

During lessons I often notice that participants do not know what to do with the instruction, "Please stay loose and relaxed!" If they were able to move in a relaxed way they would not be taking the course! Only a few people know intuitively how to do this. That's why I try to give new associations to the term "relaxation." But how can one be active and at the same time use the muscles in a way that keeps them relaxed? Here "muscle gliding" can be very helpful. It is a good example of how an image (ideo) which we have of the muscle can turn into movement (kinesis). Seals, dolphins and otters wonderfully demonstrate the use of gliding muscle fibers. I recommend a visit to the zoo or aquarium for closer inspection.

Muscles are made of bundles of fibers, which are the cells of the muscle. The fibers are made of parallel strands of filaments, long chains of proteins arranged in segmented and orderly fashion. When a muscle contracts, the proteins do not curl or bunch up, they slide into each other. You can compare the action to pushing the teeth of two combs into each other. The combs get closer, but the teeth do not shorten in the  process. This is a very useful image: When a muscle shortens, there is no shortening from the point of view of the proteins. What takes place is a sliding action.

## muscle sliding in the upper arm

Let us assume two different aspects of the function of a muscle—tension and gliding—and feel what kind of influence focusing on one of these aspects has on our movement.

1.  Put your left hand on your right upper arm muscle and visualize the tensing and relaxing of the muscle. Tense the upper arm muscle, bend the elbow, and stretch it again. Repeat five to eight times.

2. Now put the right hand on the left upper arm muscle. Visualize the muscle filaments sliding into each other when bending the elbow and sliding out again when stretching it. Focus your awareness on the muscle as if you were right in the middle of it.

Repeat, slowly, ten times.

Now let the arms hang by your side and compare the feeling in the arms and shoulders. Bend both elbows — which is easier? Which can bend further?

## movement in every cell

We develop a lot of strength and harmonious movement when we become aware that we have contractible fibers in every cell of our body. It is not as if our skeletal muscles alone are responsible for our movement and have to drag the rest of the body along with them. Even neurons and connective tissue cells have muscle fibers that are responsible for the transport system inside the cell.

Imagine that every cell is involved in our movement. All cells are elastic and have the ability to contract and relax. Start to lift your arms and shoulders with this feeling of complete mobility, and let them sink down again.

Then include the back, the neck, and the head in the vision of contracting and relaxing cells—every cell has contracting power, every cell is a muscle. Alternate, placing an emphasis on contraction and relaxation. The feeling starts to spread over the whole body—into the pelvis and the legs and feet. No movement can exhaust us. We can extend ourselves in space in all directions with the same lightness. It is truly a delight to feel that we have strength for movement and flexibility throughout our body.

After having explored this feeling for a while, try to execute a movement from daily life (getting up, sitting down, lifting a plate) without losing the feeling of whole body movement. Don't lift a plate with only the arm, but with the help of all the cells in the body. Even the brain and the nervous system are included in the execution of the movement—not only as the center of control but as active supporting parts.

## the trapezius

The trapezius is a key muscle for free–breathing movement. In its ideal state it produces relaxed movement, free breathing, a good posture, and inner peace. It was originally a gill–lifting muscle, a pure head muscle, and it seems that the trapezius likes to withdraw to its place of origin and drags the whole shoulder girdle with it. The famous knot in the shoulder mostly stems from this muscle.

It is separated into descending, ascending, and horizontal parts. The descending part starts at the back of the head at the spinous processes of the cervical spine and stretches in an elegant loop to the outer part of the collarbone and the shoulder blade. The trapezius can lift the shoulder blade and helps with its rotating. The horizontal part reaches from the spinous processeses of the thoracic spine to the spine of the scapula and can contract the

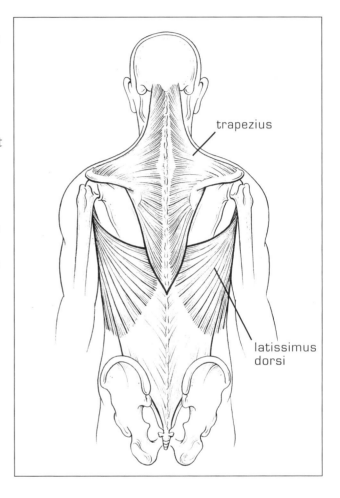

shoulder blades. The ascending part reaches from the lower spine to the spine of the scapula (see also page 41). It pulls the shoulder blade downwards and also takes part in its rotation, together with the serratus anterior muscle a movement that is essential in lifting the arm over 90 degrees (see page 52).

If there is a chronic shortening of the trapezius the shoulder blade is permanently turned in such a way that the shoulder joint is pointing upwards. The upper inner corner of the shoulder blades pulled towards the spine. Unfortunately this posture pattern is to be found quite often. If the trapezius is flacid, the opposite happens—the socket of the shoulder joint points downwards. Without the stabilizing effect of the trapezius and the serratus anterior muscle we would be unable to lift the arm at all. Since the arm is much heavier than the shoulder blade, it would already be pressed down when only lifting the arm a little. The illustration shows how the trapezius is involved in the rotation of the shoulder blade.

Interestingly, the trapezius is its own antagonist: it pulls the shoulder blade upwards, but also downwards. All the parts taken together look like a kite. This also makes for a nice image: the trapezius as a kite fluttering in the wind.

The trapezius is a key muscle for relaxation. It is one of the first muscles to get tense under stress, but when it is relaxed it has a very beneficial effect on our mental state.

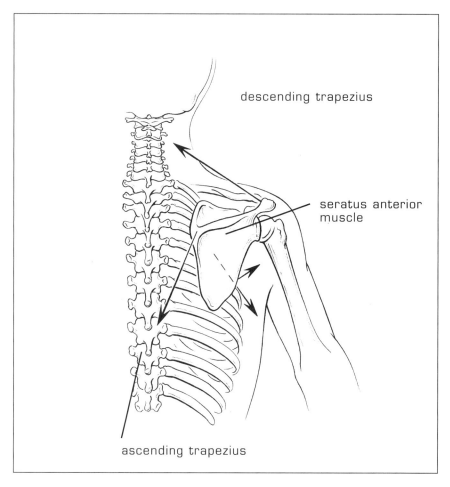

descending trapezius

seratus anterior muscle

ascending trapezius

Inner peace is one of the most important conditions for truly relaxing the trapezius.

Usually we hold our head too far forward in relationship to the spine. This means a lot of extra work for the trapezius, which has to hold the head from falling forward. If the trapezius is relaxed, the head automatically centers on the spine and this is very helpful to the cervical spine. Artificially pulling back the head doesn't help, though. The balance of the trapezius has to happen from the inside.

Many directions of flows can be experienced in the body. One can visualize them as arrows in the muscles that indicate a thrust or current. This is a concept that is somewhat explored both in ideokinesis and BMC. In ideokinesis they are called "lines of movement" in BMC they are called "currents."

### currents of the trapezius

The current of the trapezius reveals itself in its upward and downward movements in opposite directions (see diagram). The descending part of the trapezius can be visualized as a flow from the back of the head down and outwards to the collarbone and shoulder blade or feel like a ballroom dress, which spreads out on the upper back.

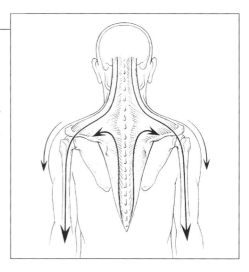

The lower part of the trapezius streams like a water fountain from the middle of the spine

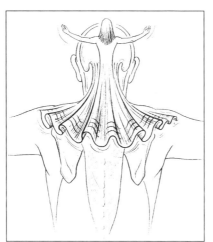

upward towards the spine of the scapula. It is especially beneficial to get the feel of these ascending currents—it can cause an immediate relaxation of the lower part of the muscle.

## stroking the trapezius

A partner can help you to feel the currents in the trapezius and the whole back by stroking his or her hands over your back. During the exercise you don't have to stay with a particular direction or follow the currents, but can discover with the hands what feels pleasant.

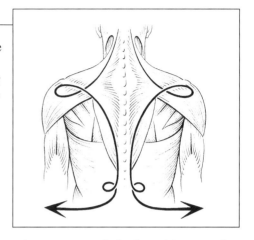

The picture shows a possible course over the trapezius and the back muscles. The wiping down should be done with a lot of verve and awareness of the breathing. During the wiping down, slowly exhale and imagine that the trapezius is sinking down to the heels.

In the following experiment we will activate the ascending trapezius. It is much weaker than the descending trapezius. A good balance between the ascending and the descending parts is an important condition for relaxed shoulders. This is also true of other muscles that lower the shoulder blade like the latissimus dorsi, the lower part of the serratus anterior muscle, and parts of the pectoralis major and minor. These will also be used in the following exercise, which has a very positive effect on shoulder balance.

## pushing the door and table push-ups

Find a door that is not too high, and put your right hand on the upper edge of the door. Lift the lcft shoulder and the shoulder blade. While pulling down with the right hand on the door, lower the shoulder again. Repeat this about three times. During this movement you may feel an active muscle at the bottom of your shoulder: this is the ascending part of the trapezius. If there is no suitable door edge, you can use anything stable which has the approximate height of your out-stretched arm. The step of a winding staircase or a cupboard door can also be used. Repeat on the other side.

If you cannot find anything suitable, you can do table push-ups.

Press both hands on the table and push up. Then let your spine sink between the shoulder blades. Press the shoulders downwards and lift the spine up again, pushing with both hands with equal strength. Repeat this about five times and try to visualize the lenthening action of the ascending fibers of the trapezius during the lowering phase. While pressing downwards the descending fibres lengthen. The movement should be done slowly and with relaxed breathing.

# active muscle elongation

Some of the exercises in this book are so–called "active muscle elongation" (AE) exercises. In active elongation the muscle acts as a brake. When putting a sleeping baby down into its crib, most of our arm and back muscles have to slowly elongate for the baby to be put down gently. This takes strength. If the muscles were to suddenly go limp, the child would not be put down very gently and the resultant screaming would remind us that we have failed to use the active elongation of the muscle (also called "eccentric action"). Active elongation greatly strengthens the muscles. This is good news for mothers and fathers who do not have time to  go to the fitness center but spend their time cradling their young children. AE exercises have the advantage that they show the muscle how to create stretch and strength at the same time.

## office chair, trapezius: active elongation

A typical office chair with a single connection between seat and back is perfect for this exercise. Our goal is to experience the rotation of the shoulder blade on the thorax, which is mainly produced by the trapezius, or from another point of view—the thorax rotating on the shoulder blade.

Sit on the chair and hold the connective part of the chair behind your back with your right hand and bend your head carefully to the left. Be careful—many of us are so tense in this area that it only needs a very small movement to reach the limit of elongation. Daily, careful exercising is preferable to a radical cure.

Because we are holding on to the chair, the shoulder can't move upwards. If this was not the case, the trapezius would not be stretched. Visualize the descending trapezius fibers sliding apart from each other, and the thorax rotating to underneath the shoulder blade. Carefully lift your head back up, rotating the thorax in the opposite direction. It can help to pull on the chair with your hand.

Repeat the movement three times.

Before changing sides, hold your arms up in the air and compare them.

If there isn't an appropriate chair, you can also do the exercise standing up by holding on to a door handle behind you. (Don't forget to hang up a notice on the other side of the door: "Exercise in process—do not enter!")

## the rhomboids

Via the rhomboid major and minor, the inner edge of the shoulder blade hangs from the spinous processes of the upper spine. Their task, together with the serratus anterior and the teres major, is to optimize the positioning of the shoulder blade for every arm movement. The rhomboid is a counter to the teres major, which would—without the pull of the rhomboid—pull the shoulder blade to the arm. Some people have a tendency to carry the shoulder blades too high up on the back which hampers the function of this muscle. If our upper body posture is not sufficiently elevated and the shoulders are rounded, the rhomboid has to work to stop the shoulder blades from turning outwards, and so they grow tired and cannot fulfill their task properly. This reveals itself in tension between the shoulder blades.

The horizontal fibers of the trapezius lie on the rhomboid. They also connect the spinous processes of the spine with the shoulder blade, specifically to the spine of the scapula. When lifting the arms these muscles as well as the levator scapulae work eccentrically to stabilize the shoulder blade. Visualize this lengthening action when you lift your arms to create a sense of space between the shoulder blades.

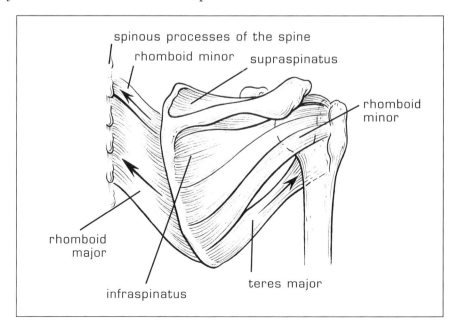

spinous processes of the spine

rhomboid minor    supraspinatus

rhomboid minor

rhomboid major

infraspinatus

teres major

A whole chain of muscles begins with the rhomboid, which continues on to the serratus anterior muscle, and the external oblique muscle, right to the front of the pelvis. This chain is important for our posture, because it helps to center the thorax on top of the pelvis.

Also, the exercises for the shoulder blade (see pages 26–28) are very helpful for loosening the rhomboid.

In the following exercise we will look at tension between the shoulder blades. The exercise will be done with a Thera-Band® (see page 108).

It is important to remember that in these exercises you can choose whatever intensity of stretching you are comfortable with.

### no more pain in the shoulder blades

During this exercise we will concentrate on the shoulder blades and the muscles between them. These are the rhomboid and the horizontal part of the trapezius.

Place the Thera-Band® across the upper back and hold both ends in your hands. Turn your arms outward and push them against the band; at the same time bend the knees and spine. Try to pull the shoulder blades apart. You will probably already feel the rhomboids quite clearly—ideally a feeling of "healthy" pain, as if those muscles have been waiting since the beginning of time for this moment! Don't overdo it—and keep breathing! Stretch the legs and spine and bring the shoulder blades towards each other again.

Repeat this movement two or three times.

Then put the band down and take in the liberated sensation between the shoulder blades.

## the serratus anterior muscle

The serratus anterior muscle starts at the upper eight ribs, crosses under the shoulder blade, and ends at its inner edge. If the lower part of the serratus anterior muscle shortens, then the shoulder blade is turned so that the socket of the shoulder joint points upwards. As mentioned already, this muscle is what makes lifting of the arm more than 90–degrees possible. In this job it is supported by the trapezius (see page 44). The situation is like a big flywheel, which is pushed from different sides at the same time. The strength of the different "flywheel" muscles is very important, but usually there is an over–emphasis on the descending part of the trapezius; the ascending part and the serratus anterior muscle are neglected during rotation.

The upper part of the serratus anterior muscle aids with shoulder rotation in the other direction to bring the shoulder socket facing downwards. When lowering the arm, all the muscles that rotated the shoulder blade with concentric action are elongated—activated eccentrically. To visualize this is very helpful, because we can rely on a lot of different muscles at the same time. The following exercise helps with this.

### the Statue of Liberty lowers her arm

Stand up and take a book in your hand. Lift your right arm up while holding the book or a similar object. The resulting position is similar to that of the Statue of Liberty in New York. Now lower the stretched arm very slowly—I emphasize slowly. Feel the rotation of the shoulder blade as if it were rolling sideways. Repeat this movement twice.

Put the book away and compare the shoulders. Perhaps you can feel that something has changed regarding the position of the shoulder blade. It is lower and the shoulder feels more relaxed.

Now repeat the exercise with the other arm.

Are there muscles that are elongated when lifting the arm? Yes: the rhomboid, the levator scapulae, the upper parts of the

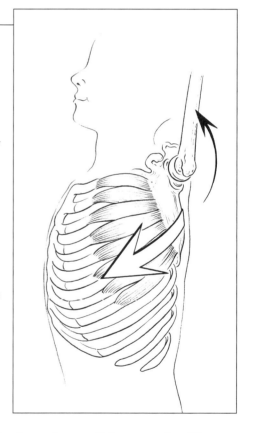

serratus anterior muscle, and the horizontal part of the trapezius. To simplify, we will only concentrate on the the rhomboids and the levator scapulae, because these two especially are in need of elongation.

## elongation when lifting the arm

Lift both arms straight up in the air and imagine that the space between the shoulder blades is enlarged. Hold the arms in this position for a while and visualize the elongation of the levator scapulae and rhomboids. Let the arms bend and slowly come down. Once again lift the arms while concentrating on the space between the shoulder blades. If you get the feeling that it tightens up, this means that you are pulling the shoulders back and pushing the head forwards. To avoid this, make sure you do not change the position of the head while lifting the arms

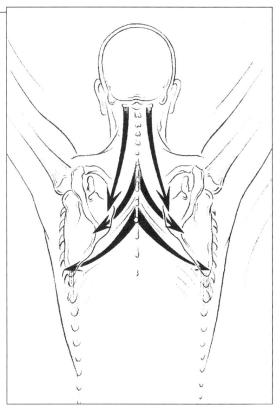

## the levator scapulae

The levator scapula is a renegade serratus anterior muscle. The serratus anterior muscle goes from the shoulder blade to the ribs, the levator scapulae from the shoulder blade to the neck. Originally we had ribs on our neck; we lost them so that we could better turn our head—an advantage when we want to quickly see what made that creaky noise behind us!

The levator scapulae goes from the inner edge of the shoulder blades to where those ribs used to be, to the front of the transverse processes of the cervical vertebras one to four. Since many people carry their shoulder blades too high, this muscle is often shortened and tense.

### touching the levator scapulae

Touch the mastoid process (a very prominent bone) which is behind the ear lobe. Right underneath it is the mastoid of the top vertebra. This spot may be quite painful. When sliding your finger down, you may discover further painful spots. In this area, under many layers of muscle, the transverse processes of the cervical vertebras can be found. Visualize the levator scapulae running from the upper four transverse processes to the inner upper edge of the shoulder blade.

The origin of the levator scapulae at the shoulder blade can barely be felt when our arms are hanging by our side, since it is covered by the trapezius. If we lean our elbows on the table, the shoulder blade glides upwards. Then the descending trapezius is somewhat relaxed and we can better touch the upper edge of the shoulder blade.

Touch the left shoulder blade at the base of the neck with the right hand. Slide your fingers along the inner edge of the shoulder blade upwards till you come to the origin of the levator scapulae. Be careful, because a lot of painful spots and muscle knots can be found in this area.

Now visualize an ascending current through the levator scapulae and a descending one through the trapezius (an image adapted from BMC®). Travel with your fingers from the shoulder blade to the upper transverse processes of the spine, and from the back of the head along the trapezius downward to the acromion. Repeat on the other side.

### the neck hangs from the shoulder blade

The thorax of quadrupeds hangs from the top of the serratus muscle on the shoulder blades. Get onto "all fours" where you can lower and lift your thorax to exercise the serratus muscle.

The levator scapula is also a serratus muscle. We can imagine how the upper four vertebras via the levator scapulae hang from the shoulder blades. Lowering the head and neck elongates the levator scapulae and lifting them shortens it. Can you also visualize this image while standing up? This gives the neck a feeling of lengthening and lightness.

## the triangular or deltoid muscle

The triangular or deltoid muscle covers the shoulder joint like a cap. It corresponds to the gluteus maximus muscle on the pelvis. The deltoid originates at the spine of the scapula, the acromion, and from the collarbone and runs to the middle of the upper arm. It consists of front, middle, and back parts. The deltoid lifts the arm sideways, and also to the front, different parts of it being used for both movements. It also helps with the inward and outward rotation of the arm. Luckily it is seldom part of the tension pattern in the shoulders, which is why its cooperation with other shoulder muscles is vital. Visualize it flowing from the acromion to the upper arm.

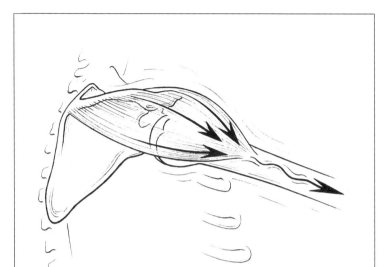

## lifting the arm with the deltoid

Put your left hand on the right deltoid and exhale through the muscle, from the collarbone and the shoulder blade right down to the middle of the upper arm. Slowly lift your right arm sideways, while visualizing a flow through the muscle, until the arm points diagonally upward.

Now lower the arm and maintain the same direction of flow.

Repeat three times.

Compare the left and the right deltoid by letting the arms hang by your side after the exercise.

Lift both arms sideways with your eyes closed and see which side is easier to move. Even if you do not feel a difference, on opening your eyes you might notice that the arm on this side is held higher up. This shows that visualizing flow improves flexibility.

Now repeat the exercise on the other side.

Often the flow or current of one muscle continues into another. The current of the descending trapezius continues into the deltoid. The situation is similar to a waterfall that falls over some steps. In this case the steps are the collarbone and the shoulder blade, which is where the two muscles are attached. On top of these two bones flows the trapezius and below the deltoid.

### the combined
### deltoid-trapezius currents

Glide your hand down the side of the back of the head along the trapezius to the acromion. From there continue to the middle of the upper arm. Here the deltoid ends. This stroking can be done while holding the arm up and to the side.

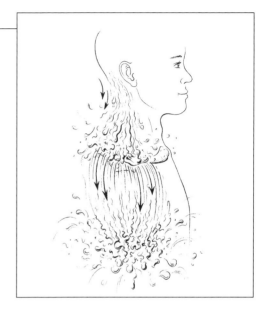

## arm rotators

Different muscles that rotate the arm both inward and outward are attached to the shoulder blade. They are called the rotator cuff muscles, even though their main task is to stabilize the shoulder joint. Accordingly, their currents converge in the middle of the shoulder blade. The deltoid tends to pull the upper arm upward out of the shoulder joint when we lift the arm. The cuff muscles infraspinatus, the teres minor, and the subscapularis muscle take care of a stabilizing counter rotation.

The subscapularis lies, as its name indicates, under the shoulder blade and provides a pleasant gliding surface for its movements. The subscapularis sits, like the filling in a sandwich, between the shoulder blade and the thorax and turns the arm inwards. It is supported in its activity by the teres major, which is attached to the backside of the shoulder blade. This muscle is the slightly short brother of the latissimus dorsi, but supports it energetically in the pulling down of the arm. The supraspinatus lies in the valley, up on the spine of the scapula, and makes sure that the head of the upper arm sits firmly in its socket. Unfortunately the supraspinatus overdoes it sometimes in its eagerness to hold the joint and gets tense. When lifting the arm, visualize the descending currents of the deltoid and the ascending currents of the supraspinatus at the same time. This aids in optimally relaxed coordination during the lifting of the arm.

## good old shoulder gymnastics

In this exercise we will activate almost all the shoulder muscles, especially the rotators.

Put your fingers on top of one shoulder and make a big circular movement in one direction with the elbow of the same arm.

After having circled the elbow about five times, stretch the arm and make big circles with the hand.

Now put the fingers back on the shoulder and make circles in the other direction five times. Then stretch the arm and circle the hand five times.

Repeat the exercise on the other side.

## waving with the arm rotators

I recommend you use air-filled balls of 5–10 cm (2 to 4 inches) in diameter for this exercise (see page 108). The balls are used as ball bearings between the arms and the floor. This provides an increase in the range of movement.

Lie down on your back. Put the balls underneath the middle of your upper arms. Place a small cushion under your head. Rest the elbows at a 90–degree angle, and point the lower arms at the ceiling.

To loosen the inward rotators (subscapularis, teres major), slowly rotate the arms outwards—the back of the hands get closer to the floor. Think of the shoulder blades sinking to the floor. When the hands can't go any lower, make small, snaky movements with the spine.

Move the hands upwards again and rotate the arms the other way. Now the palms face the floor, the upper arm bone rotates inwards—now we are elongating the external rotators (infraspinatus, teres minor). Again, when the hands can't move further, make small snake-like movements with the spine.

Repeat this slow motion, hand-waving movement five times. Try to visualize which muscles are shortened and which ones are lengthened as you proceed.

Slowly lift the hands up again, put the balls away, and observe what has changed in the shoulders.

This exercise can also be done with small weights held in the hand. It is important to proceed slowly and stop immediately if there is any pain.

## the major and minor pectorals

The pectoralis major is attached to the upper arm and continues like a wide open fan to the collar and breastbone, and to the upper ribs. It is even connected to the rectus sheath, the connective tissue sheath of the rectus abdominis muscle. It pulls the arm powerfully toward the front of the body, a movement typical to boxing. Because its fibers run in different ascending and descending diagonals, it can move the arm both horizontally and up and down. It likes to work together with other muscles of the shoulder girdle to generate strong and spacious movements. In gymnastics it can unfold its full potential—when doing pull-ups and crawling it cooperates with the latissimus dorsi. Interestingly, it is twisted just before its attachment to the upper arm. This makes sure that the length of the fibers of the pectoralis doesn't vary too much in the different arm positions.

In its cramped state it is unfortunately responsible, together with the pectoralis minor, for forward rounded shoulders. Through this the center of gravity is moved away from its alignment over the pelvis and burdens the back muscles with too much work. The neck muscles strain to provide the forward-falling shoulders with a counterweight.

It sometimes seems as if the pectoral muscles are trying to place our shoulders in front of our heart like two sliding doors to emotionally protect us. Accordingly we may feel naked when the pectoralis has been lengthened and the breastbone sticks out in all its glory.

This is a difficulty found when changing a pattern of muscle–shortening: are we emotionally ready to be open in this area? For many, this is fraught with anxiety and that is why one often falls back into the old posture pattern after an exercise. But it is worth sticking at it. The upper back will reward your perseverance with suppleness.

The pectoralis minor originates from the second to fifth rib and continues to the coracoid process (see page 36). It can lower the shoulder blade and is a kind of frontal connector to the horizontal part of the trapezius. Together they enable a solid positioning of the shoulder blade. When you vigorously push down the shoulder blade you can feel the pectoralis minor underneath the collarbone on the thorax.

## muscle sliding in the pectoralis major

Lift the left arm. Put the palm of the right hand on the pectoralis major between breastbone, collarbone, and shoulders.

Feel your breathing in the muscle.

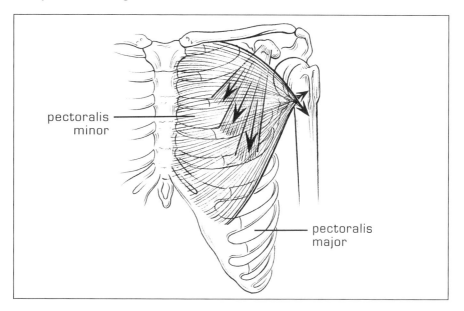

pectoralis minor

pectoralis major

Now move the arm in front of your body, until the elbow comes to lie almost in front of the breastbone. Feel how the pectoralis major gets thicker as the filaments slide into each other.

Move the arm outwards again—now the filaments slide away from each other.

Repeat this movement a few times, still feeling your breathing in the muscle. Inhale and visualize the filaments sliding together; exhale and imagine them sliding apart.

Repeat this movement about ten times.

Compare the feeling in both shoulders and in the pectorals before exercising on the other side of the body.

Perhaps you can feel more space in the left upper thorax area. Has your breathing changed?

## currents in the pectorals

Lie down on your back and feel your shoulders lying on the ground. Are they lying a little off the ground? Does the pectoralis feel a bit tight?

Visualize the fan-like pectoralis major with its attachments to the collarbone, the breastbone and the rectus sheath.

Hold your arms up vertically, perpendicular to the breastbone. Let them sink down slowly sideways and imagine how the pectoralis major is lengthening. Feel the quality of this movement: is it flowing, is there tension?

Lift the arms into the air again. As they sink, visualize how the pectoralis major is elongated. It fans out in the direction of the upper arm. Underneath it lies the pectoralis minor. Can you feel its current from the coracoid to the upper ribs?

Repeat this movement again. How does it feel now? How far can you let the arms sink down? Are the shoulders now lying more solidly on the ground than before?

## the latissimus dorsi

The latissimus dorsi is the biggest muscle in the body. It is very important for the alignment of the shoulder girdle and the well-being of the entire back. It is attached to the small tuberosity on the front of the upper arm bone. Its origins are numerous. The latissimus dorsi originates from the thoracolumbar fascia, between the spinous processes of the sixth thoracic vertebra, right to the sacrum; also on the ninth to twelfth ribs, and on the last third of the iliac crest. The thoracolumbar fascia is a thick slab of connective tissue that covers and strengthens the lower part of the back. If this fascia is tight, it can cause back pain. This muscle connects the sacrum and the iliac crest with the front part of the arm. That's why arm movements and the state of the lower back are inescapably connected to each other.

The latissimus dorsi is the cross-country muscle par excellence, since it can pull the arms behind the body and rotate them inwards. It also actively helps with climbing and swimming. It is an important stabilizer of the shoulder joint and can take over the task of antagonist to the anterior deltoid and the pectoralis major. By adding this muscle to the internal image of our body, we can get a new feeling of support for the arms in all our movements.

If the latissimus dorsi is tight, the pelvis is tipped forward when lifting the arm and the the lumbar spine will become hollowed. This is a pattern that is seen often. In this condition exercise involving a lot of arm movement can be harmful to the shoulders and the back.

## becoming aware of the latissimus

This is an exercise to be done in pairs.

Stand behind your partner, who should raise his or her arms. Touch the anterior of the upper arm bone close to the shoulder joint with your fingers. Then stroke down to the lower tip of the shoulder blade and to the sixth/seventh spinous process of the thoracic spine. With your thumbs on the spinous processes, stroke with widely fanned hands downward to the iliac crest, then, narrowing your hands again, continue to the sacrum. This way we touch the whole of the latissimus dorsi.

## the currents of the latissimus dorsi

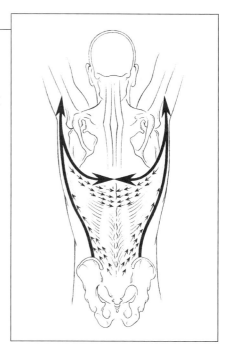

With all exercises it is helpful to visualize the currents, the flowing direction, of the latissimus dorsi. Especially when lifting and lowering the arms—a movement often used in everyday life—visualizing the lines-of-movement of this muscle is very useful. The lower fibers of the latissimus dorsi, which originate at the iliac crest, and those which come from the sacrum and the lumbar region, all flow in a current upwards to the arm. The fibers that go from the upper arm over the lower shoulder angle to the sixth thoracic vertebra stream in the opposite direction, towards the spine. It feels as if the outer and lower back area can only become relaxed if the middle is "tied up." When one has mastered the currents a bit, one gets the feeling that the arms are sitting on the latissimus, like two candles resting in a candle holder.

## active elongation of the latissimus dorsi

Lie down on a comfortable mat. Stretch the legs out or bend them with the feet resting on the ground. Visualize the latissimus dorsi as a huge silk cloth (see drawing) that is sinking to the ground with a fluttering movement.

Stretch your arms up, and let them sink down slowly next to the head. Imagine that the muscle is a huge piece of chewing gum which is stretching from the lower back and the back of the pelvis to the front of the upper arm.

Maybe you can feel the pull of the latissimus dorsi on a certain part of the back. Try to target and loosen this spot with your imagination and breathing.

Repeat this movement five times. You can also breathe into the muscle and visualize the sliding apart of the muscle fibers.

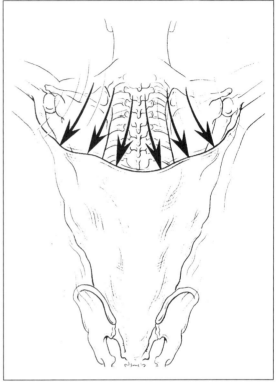

## latissimus stretching with a band

Attach a long medium-strong Thera-Band® to something stable and tie a knot so there is a loop. Hold the band with both hands and bend down a bit. This exercise can also be done with a partner.

Bend your knees. The band should not be stretched too much, just as far as you feel a pleasant pull in the back and in the shoulders. If you are with a partner, make sure that you are not both pulling on the band at the same time but have a playful back and forth action.

Move the back in different ways, and sigh a bit if you like. Exhale and give some weight over to the band. Don't hold the neck stiffly, but let the head hang and swing a little bit. Stay active in the pelvis and legs. Also try to rotate the trunk and to let the shoulder blades slide along the back.

In between, allow the upper body to hang completely free and use the elasticity of the band to loosen the shoulders.

Now pull the band to your back, and move it forward again slowly. If you bend your arms, then the extensor of the elbow gets exercised. If you try to pull the band down and back with stretched out arms, then the latissimus dorsi is exercised. While slowly moving the arms forward again, the latissimus dorsi and the teres major have to put on the brakes. That's why you may feel some activity in the lateral part of the back. Can this be felt equally strongly on both sides?

Repeat this movement five times.

Slowly stand up and observe what has changed in the posture of the shoulders.

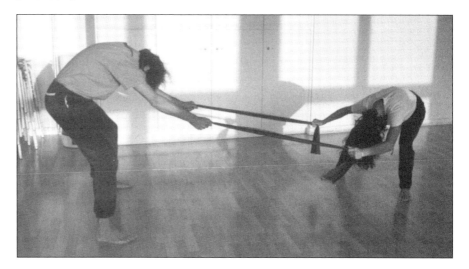

# 5  Organ Relaxation

**B**ecause every part of the body can get tense—right down to single cells—it is important to know a broad spectrum of remedies. It is with this that the perception of the holistic functioning of the body begins. When we have mastered exercising with imagery, we can reach all areas of the body—including the organs—and, depending on what's needed, activate or relax them.

It is important that every organ moves three-dimensionally, and that it fully takes up the space allocated to it.  Organs can be metaphorically seen as either muscle-tubes (digestion organs), water balloons (liver) or muscular spunges (lungs, spleen, thymus gland).

The capabilities of the organs are very impressive. A normal muscle is exhausted after 10 minutes of non–stop activity, and needs thirty minutes of rest afterward. If the heart had similar capabilities, our life expectancy wouldn't exactly be fabulous. Organ movement cannot be compared to the linear movement of muscles, but nevertheless they are truly amazing: who can expand their arm to twice its size? Yet, the spleen can expand like a sponge to twice its size. The strongest muscle in the body is also an organ: the uterus. Unfortunately, men don't have anything similar to offer, except the bladder, which is lined with a triple layer of muscle.

An important goal of this training is to give the organs the experience of being in varied positions. Instead of being layered the same way all the time, they can experience the vertical and horizontal from time to time. For example, rolling on the floor is very enlivening for the organs and improves circulation and detoxification.

Once one has experienced the degree to which the organs can enable a grounding and relaxed uplifting of the posture, one wonders why in the schooling of posture rarely a word is said about the importance of the organs.

To truly feel the organs brings a wider perception of space as well as a deep relaxation—a feeling of being with oneself. When we relax the organs, we can feel a distancing from our daily troubles. It is a feeling of letting go, an important step on the path of life. Problems just bounce off us, and it becomes difficult to ponder all one's little difficulties and hurts—they no longer seem very relevant.

Everybody feels this when I ask them, after having done an organ exercise during a workshop, "Everyone, try now to think about a problem." The participants experience that if they change their physical state, and their perception of the body, this also changes the content of their thoughts.

I believe problems are overcome more easily in this state because they are perceived in a more objective light.

### the lung-heart connection

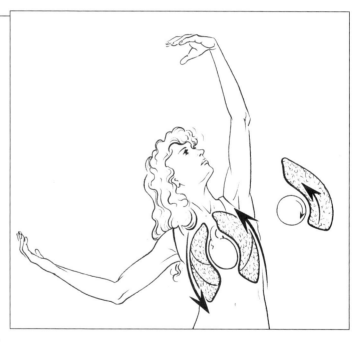

The lungs and the heart have a lot to do with the posture of the upper body and therefore with the state of the neck and shoulders. If we have a slack, bent posture in the upper body, both lobes of the lungs are shielding the heart—like an eclipse of the sun. Our heart is physically and emotionally cramped in its expression.

In the following way the space around the heart can be developed positively. Imagine that your heart and the neighbouring lung constitute a ball and socket-joint. The heart represents the ball, and the lungs represent the socket. Both joint surfaces are well lubricated and allow three-dimensional movement.

Stretch the left arm out in front of you and imagine the lung gliding in front of and around the heart—the socket turning around the ball. Move the arm back again and visualize how the socket moves back again around the heart. At this point the heart, the ball of the joint, moves a little in the direction of the breastbone. Exercise this movement upwards and downwards as well. Stretch your left arm upwards, and the lung glides up over the heart. Let the arm come down, and the lung glides over the heart downward. Repeat this movement a few times.

Compare both sides of the upper body before you repeat the exercise on the other side.

## the lungs are obscured by clouds

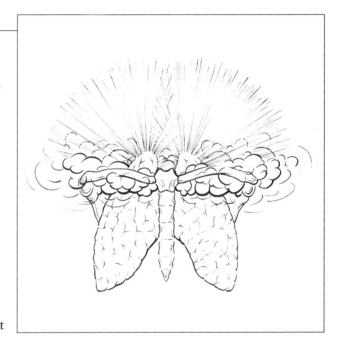

Imagine the collarbone, the breastbone, and the shoulderblade as a ring of clouds that softly encompasses the lungs. Lift up the shoulder-girdle so that the lungs disappear into the depths of the clouds. Lower the shoulders and imagine the lungs sticking out of the clouds like mountain tops in the sunlight. Repeat this movement a few times, and feel how the lungs get a little further out of this ring of clouds with each movement.

The lungs are very important to the posture and looseness of the shoulders and neck. If the lungs do not fill out the space allocated to them, and if they are a little atrophied, then the shoulder and neck muscles have to compensate, and this causes tension. This is often a cause of bad posture. It is equally important that the lungs glide smoothly within the pulmonary pleura during inhalation and exhalation. When I touch the shoulders of a client, it sometimes feels as if the lungs have retracted somewhat; to my inner eye it looks as if the waves (the inhaling and exhaling) are no longer flooding the beach completely.

### the apex of the lungs as a soft nose

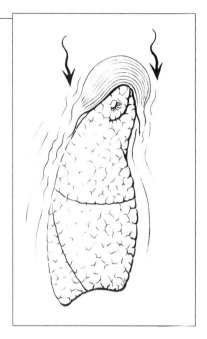

Put your left hand on your right shoulder and visualize the position of the apex of the lung beneath your hand. This apex protrudes like a seal's wet nose over the first rib (images are a matter of personal taste!) Imagine how the shoulder muscles (trapezius) lie on the apex of the lungs and relax like a piece of melting cheese.

The lung contains a million small bubble–like chambers where the exchange of gases takes place. These spheres are called alveoli. Around the alveoli and the bronchi, transporting the air to and fro, are wound small, smooth muscle ribbons, like Christmas baubles, around which are wrapped golden ribbons—except that they are very elastic.

First, circle your right shoulder and imagine that the apex of the lung itself could trigger this movement. Then change the direction of the circling and feel how the soft, elastic content of the shoulder triggers the movement.

Put your hand on the middle lobe of the lung and try to lift the lung a little, and then lower it again. The thorax and shoulders move as well, but the trigger of the movement comes from the lung.

Lay your hand on the lower lobe of the lung. It can be found mainly close to the back and is therefore more difficult to touch. Guide your breathing to the lower lobe of the lung; visualize its position on the diaphragm. While inhaling, its underside expands like a broad bottom on the diaphragm. While exhaling it contracts again. Try to lift the apex of the lung a bit, and then lower it again.

Now compare your shoulders. Can you feel the difference?

Do the same exercise with the other side, although on the left side there isn't a separate middle lobe.

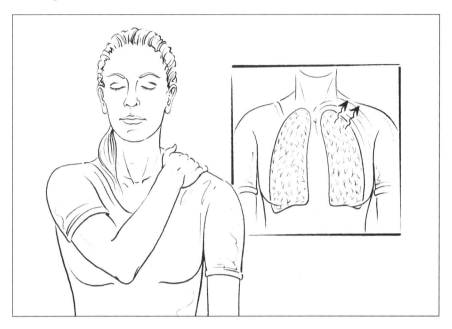

## heart or brain

In *The Wizard of Oz* there is a heated discussion between the Scarecrow and the Tinman. The Tinman would very much like to have a heart, and the Scarecrow a brain. The Tinman says, "I've had a spell cast on me and now I am made completely of tin. I am so lonely, because somebody who doesn't have a heart can't love."

The Scarecrow retorts, "I will ask for a brain, since a dummy wouldn't even know what to do with a heart."

The Tinman replies, "I once had a heart and a brain—I have had both. I would rather have a heart, since a brain doesn't make you happy."

Luckily we do not have to decide between a heart and a brain. The question is only whether they are working harmoniously together, supporting each other—or whether one of them dominates.

There is, though, a third fellow to be reckoned with—the belly. Here lies the center of the body, the Hara, which you may know from various meditation techniques.

Anatomically we can find the "enteric brain," or the intestinal brain, in the wall of the gut, which has aroused recent scientific interest. In the intestinal wall there is a two-layered neuroplexus which is so extensive that it can be looked on virtually as a brain in its own right. It is connected with the rest of the body through an important nerve, the vagus. The enteric brain combines many aspects of the central nervous system. It has as many neurons as the spinal cord and produces the same neurotransmitters and hormones as the brain. The vagus influences our emotions through its connections in the brain and has even been proposed as the site of an implant to ward off anxiety. A less invasive technique is the use of organ exercises to balance the enteric brain with the heart and head-brain.

In daily life many decisions are taken from "the gut." We sometimes do things because they "feel" right—and then the head–brain later finds a justification for our action. But the impulse for the decision came from our belly. The enteric brain could be called the primitive or primeval brain.

Primitive animals have only an enteric brain. It is located where it counts—in the mouth—and controls food intake. With humans the enteric brain is still there where the nutrients are absorbed, in the intestines—nothing is supposed to get into the system that is not good for it.

Life situations need to be digested too, and if they are unpalatable we feel it in the belly—our digestion doesn't work properly, we don't feel well. If the enteric brain is not well, the head-brain is affected: we get in a bad mood, both our verbal and other kinds of expression become more and more negative. The reverse is also possible: when we are not able to digest something with our mind, then the enteric brain is affected. Stress causes digestion problems—the enteric brain takes hours to absorb nutrients, the head-brain wants to devour them in three minutes.

The enteric brain can be compared with the nourishing earth: it is our one constant factor while the head is making plans and analyzing situations. In the middle sits the heart, which can only manifest itself when the brain and the belly are working together harmoniously. Devotion, love, and bliss cannot be expressed in the middle of a fight between the belly and the brain.

For people with tension in the upper body it can be very helpful to discover how the health of the enteric brain affects the head–brain when the buzzing brain gets an anchor in our center. This alone can heal a lot of tension and even illness of a chronic nature. When there is calmness, the heart can beat more slowly and contribute to well–being. The dialogue between head, belly and heart enables harmony, through which the person can develop.

## visualizing the enteric brain

Lie down comfortably on a mat. To be able to feel the belly better, put a warm towel on it. Visualize the intestines and the different layers of the enteric brain—the many nerves are shining with a golden glow. Imagine that the nerves have a lot of strength and know exactly what is good for us. Breathe into and out of the enteric brain. With every breath the cells of the enteric brain shine brighter.

Feel how the back, the shoulders and the whole body relax.

## bringing energy into the belly

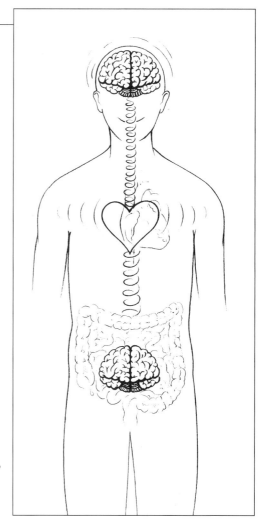

Sit on a chair with an upright and relaxed posture—feet on the floor, hands lying on the belly. Breathe a few times gently into the belly. Now imagine that energy is sinking from the head, neck and shoulders into the belly. If you can't imagine "energy," choose a metaphor like a soft golden light that streams from the shoulders and the neck to the belly.

Concentrate on your belly and imagine it is filled with energy or light. Visualize your brain and let it relax on this new foundation of energy in the belly; it rests upon the belly-energy and even sinks downwards slightly towards the belly.

Feel the connection between the enteric brain and the head-brain, an exchange of energies that is equal in both directions, like two ascending and descending elevators next to each other. Visualize your heart in the middle of these two poles. It is floating, carried by balanced head and belly–brain energies.

Exercise this regularly—even if you only have time for five minutes. You will see that it is worth it.

# soft axes

The gut tube is a soft channel and is the main body axis in primitive animals. It begins at the mouth, the esophagus continues on to the stomach, the small and large intestines and ends at the anus. If our gut is flaccid, the neck has to compensate with added tension. If you have a stiff neck, remind yourself that not only do we have muscles and joints in our neck, but also an elastic muscular tube. If we can identify with this elastic connection between trunk and head, our neck muscles will relax.

The esophagus consists of orbicular and longitudinal muscles and it pushes the food in continuing peristaltic movements into the stomach. It lies in front of the spine and will provide elastic support for the spine under ideal circumstances and in this way relieve the back muscles.

## activating the gut tube

Imagine the the origin of the esophagus in the stomach. From there it rises like a cobra and ends in the oral cavity. It is helpful to feel the elastic roof of the mouth, the palate. When yawning we can easily feel the palate lifting. Try to keep the palate as high as you can after yawning and at the same time be aware of the anchoring of the esophagus in the stomach.

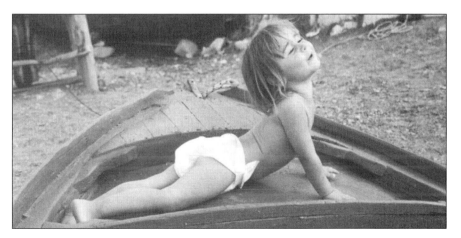

Lie on the belly and feel the movement of your breathing and the shifting of the organs in the abdominal cavity. By pressing the belly downwards we can achieve leverage into the gut and push the spine from the bottom upwards. It helps to feel like a small child that looks around itself curiously and raises itself up. You may even think of the brain as an organ floating upward.

With time you will be able to lift the head not only with muscle power but with softness.

Transfer this feeling now to sitting and standing up. Try to trigger rocking movements of the head from the stomach and gut. With every swallow, experience the strength of this soft axis. The soft palate floats upwards and the neck muscles melt down from the back of the head like warm beeswax.

### the bladder: keystone of the organ column

The organs sit like a tower of water-filled balloons on top of each other. The bladder constitutes the base of this organ tower. The bladder is a strong hollow organ that consists of three layers of muscle. It centers the pelvis and is the "keystone" of the organ column; the weight of the organs is carried to the bladder.

Lift your arms up and imagine a connection between your arms and bladder. The arms find their basis via the organ column in the keystone of the bladder. The bladder floats upwards and receives the weight of the arms.

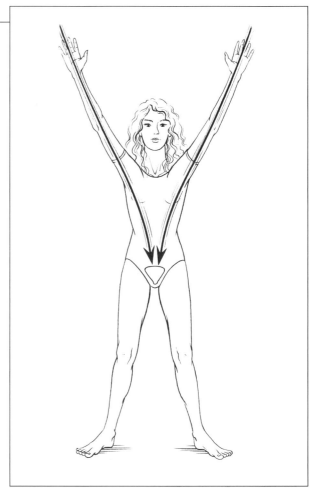

Lower the arms and feel the tension in the shoulders. Afterwards, move your arms around freely. Try to initiate these movements from the bladder.

Lack of centering and a sinking bladder can be connected with problems of the pelvic floor.

# 6 Partnering: The Relaxation Duet

**P**artner exercises are very valuable because one can work intensively with touch. For clarity's sake I will call the person who is touched "A," and the person who is touching "B."

Soft touch is worth a thousand words—and is very relaxing. The most important thing when doing touching exercises is that both A and B profit from the exercise. Person B can relax deeply too, even though he or she is not being touched. This heightens the effect of the exercise a great deal.

The primary effect of touch is always achieved through one's inner state. That is why it is important that one feels good, breathes relaxedly and sits comfortably while touching. When touching becomes too strenuous one should take a break.

The person who is being touched should immediately say if the touching becomes unpleasant in any way. Under no circumstance should person A accept an unpleasant touch from B in order not to hurt B's feelings. So stay in a dialogue: "Please touch there a bit longer. Push harder. Stop, that hurts!" One of the most important results achieved through touching is that we become more flexible and loose. How is this possible? Our whole body is represented in the brain, where there is, in fact, a map of the body. Through touching, this map can become clearer.

A comparable situation would be to drive a car in a town we do not know. To get to a particular place is not always easy—one-way streets and strange traffic situations can often cause us to despair. We need much more time to get there than we would if we knew the way already. It's even worse if we are in a car we are not familiar with, one that is bigger or smaller than our own car. Due to all these factors we take longer, make wrong turns—and get tense.

The same is true of the body. When we can't feel ourselves properly and only have a minimal experience of our body, then we have only a vague map in our nervous system. The movements of the body are restricted. If we don't have the right map of the "country" of the shoulder blade, we will not able to realize that it is being pushed slowly upwards due to tense shoulder muscles; we will also not be aware that it can only be moved in a restricted manner. If an area doesn't appear on the map, we don't consciously take it in.

Before starting the partner exercises we are going to focus some attention on the hands, since important impulses will be coming from them to our partner.

# the wrist joints

There is an astonishing connection between the wrist and the state of the shoulders and upper back. (A comparable connection exists between the tarsal bone and the lower back and the hip joint, as well as between the fingers and the shoulder blade [see page 37].) The wrist bones are made up of a lot of interconnected joints and can move three–dimensionally. The bones function like antishock pads and adjusters. If there is tension in these bones—often hardly noticeable—the corresponding shoulder and the back get tense.

The wrist consists of eight small bones with richly descriptive names that are arranged in two rows. In the row which is closer to the arm (proximal), from the thumb to the little finger there is the scaphoid, the lunate, the triquetral, and lying on the triqeutral, the pisiform bone. The pisiform bone can be felt easily on the inside of the wrist like a small knob under the skin. It is difficult to imagine that the pisiform bone corresponds to the knobbly part of the heel. The row that is closer to the palm (distal), from the thumb to the little finger is the trapezium, the trapezoid, the capitate bone and the hamate bone.

## loosening the wrist joints

Try to feel one bone after the other. The drawing on the next page will help you to remember the arrangement of these bones. When you have found them, start to massage them.

If you feel from the pisiform bone diagonally in the direction of the center of the palm you can easily feel the hamate bone, like a thick knob under the skin. Next to the hamate bone towards the middle of the hand you can find the capitate bone. If you put a finger on the back of the wrist, you can feel a little hollow on the end of the metacarpal. Here lies the capitate bone. If you bend the hand, the capitate bone pushes forward in the direction of your finger and the hollow disappears. If you move your finger a little bit further in the direction of the side of the thumb and again bend the hand, then the trapezium can be felt. Behind it, in the direction of the lower arm, there is the scaphoid bone. The lunate bone forms the central basis of the carpals and the triquetrum lies right next to it under the pisiform bone on the little finger side.

After this tour, compare the state of both your shoulders by letting your arms rest at your side. Lift both arms over your head and move them to the back. You may notice that the shoulder on the side you touched your carpal bones feels more elastic and flexible. This exercise is a fine example of how body awareness and touch can be sufficient to release tension and increase flexibility. If you lift a book with each hand, the book on the side you practiced will feel lighter. Now repeat the touching of the carpals on the other hand.

## differentiating the metacarpal bones

I highly recommend that you regularly feel and move the metacarpal bones. This exercise is doubly effective when done with some olive or sesame oil.

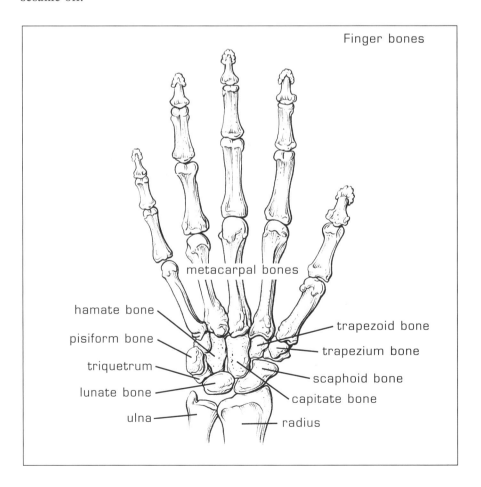

Finger bones

metacarpal bones

hamate bone

pisiform bone

triquetrum

lunate bone

ulna

trapezoid bone

trapezium bone

scaphoid bone

capitate bone

radius

The metacarpus is based on and radiates from the carpal bones.

Start from the carpal bones and feel your way over the metacarpal bones to the finger tips. When doing this try to move every metacarpal bone a little by pressing it up and down. Explore the hollows between the metacarpal bones. These spaces are filled with muscles. Try to create movement and flow in these spaces. Make sure that you don't exert yourself too much during this hand safari, and don't tense your breathing. Go to it with playful seriousness!

You may feel pain in some areas—so be careful! These exercises are especially suited to people who sit a lot at a computer or otherwise place strain on their wrists.

# roll up and roll down with the spinous processes

The alignment and the state of tension of the spinous processes located at the back of the spine are of inestimable importance for the posture and relaxation of the back and shoulders. The spine consists of 32 vertebras. Of these, 24 are independent. A vertebra consists of a body, an arch, two transverse processes and one spinous process. The only part that usually can be touched is right under the skin and is the spinous process. Because we can't see our spinous processes, we are not sufficiently aware of them.

A lot of muscles and ligaments originate on these processes. By aligning the processes, these structures are unburdened and posture improves. The relaxation of the spinous processes straightens the spine and enables the center of gravity of the shoulder girdle to sink down. This relaxes the muscles of the neck and shoulders.

If our upper body posture bends slightly forwards, the spinous process of the upper back and the muscles attached to them are under constant pull. They get tense and block the neighboring articular facets between the vertebras. Also, our spinal cord is put under more pressure, which can lead to headaches and a lack of energy.

The following exercise is done with a partner; the person touched is A, the person touching B.

## sensing the spinous processes

Person A sits on a stool with his or her back to person B, and person B touches the spinous processes one by one, starting at the pelvis. The lowest process lies a little below the iliac crest. Sometimes it is difficult to feel the spinous processes, especially if the back muscles are very tense. The touching should therefore be soft, but clear and definite.

Slowly, B moves upwards along the spine. B might notice that some of the processes are laterally displaced or are lying deeper than others.

One has to be especially careful with the cervical spine. B should try to make A aware of the positioning of his/her spinous processes in relation to each other—and A should visualize how the spinous processes align themselves to each other and that they melt away downwards.

After all the spinous processes have been touched, A slowly rolls down through the vertebra one by one, starting at the head. To do this, A bends forward, allowing the spine to curve, thus unwinding each vertebra in turn. This should be done carefully, with relaxed breathing and with concentration on the spinous processes. During the unwinding, the spinous processes fan out so that space is created between them.

The tuberosities of the ischium should be solidly anchored in the stool. B helps A to feel the processes by touching them, starting at the cervical spine.

While A presses the coccyx and the tuberosities down, he/she starts to unwind the spine again. B now starts touching above the sacrum and slowly feels the processes, adapting to A's speed of unwinding.

The most important aspect of this exercise is to feel the movement of the spinous processes.

Person A focuses on how the straightening of the spine and the situation in the shoulders is. Are they lying a bit lower, are they more relaxed?

# letting go

After a relaxing exercise the wish can easily arise that it should always be like this. Behind this lies not only the realization that relaxation connects us with an enormous potential of energy, but also the suspicion or knowledge that this state is only too easily lost in the hectic pace of daily life. We often think we need to have a grip on everything, and do not really trust the still unfamiliar feeling of letting go.

In the following exercises we will experiment with giving up and letting go, and see how this changes our experiences and our body.

### the carried shoulders (adapted from André Bernard)

This is an ideal exercise for people who like to enjoy life! It helps create the experience of walking with totally relaxed shoulders.

B puts hands under A's armpits and lifts up A's shoulders. During the whole exercise person A should allow the shoulders to be completely in the hands of B—under no circumstance should A help to lift the shoulders even though the weight of the arms and shoulders is quite substantial. If person A is ticklish, B can lift the shoulders by holding the outside of the upper arm and lifting up.In this fashion both people walk around the room for one or two minutes. Now person B slowly lets go of the shoulders. The walking and the slow letting go are very important to be able to properly experience the loosening of the shoulders.

The experiment should be repeated once more before changing partners. Depending on the weight of the shoulders, this exercise can be quite exhausting for person B, so it should only be done for one or two minutes.

### kidney lifting

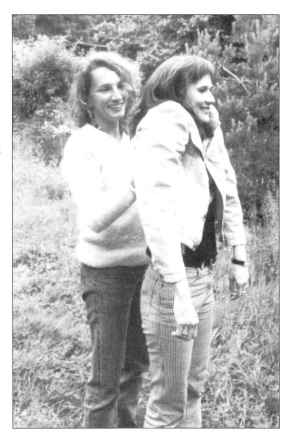

This exercise, a variation of the one on page 7, is started by charging one's hands with energy by rubbing them together and breathing into the space between them.

Then, stand behind your partner, who should be sitting comfortably, and put your hands on both his or her kidneys. Imagine that you are sending energy into the kidneys and also that you are carrying and supporting them. The feeling should be one of floating—it really is a "face-lift" for the kidneys.

## the arm game

The following experiment is about letting go of control, letting go of wanting to do everything yourself. Your partner should let one arm hang limply by the side of his or her body. You then hold the relaxed lower arm and move it in different directions—sometimes slowly, sometimes fast. You may feel that your partner is trying to help with the movement. Remind him or her to keep the arm and shoulder totally relaxed. Let the arm go without warning and test whether your partner has really relaxed the arm. Repeat this with both arms and note any difference in the looseness of the two arms.

This experiment can be done with both arms at the same time: both partners have an active and a passive arm. With your right arm move your partner's left arm, and he or she uses the right arm to move your left arm. Let go of your partner's arm in order to test whether it is relaxed.

This variation of the experiment is quite a bit more difficult because one side of the body has to stay relaxed while the other is active. Each arm should in turn be active and passive. Usually there is quite a difference between the two sides.

## moved tapping

This exercise is about increasing the sensitivity of the entire surface of the body, improving flexibility, and deepening your breathing.

Your partner relaxes into any position. Now choose an area of the body of about three to four palms width, and tap it with your finger tips, with loose wrists. Do this for about a minute and then give your partner some time to feel the effect of the tapping: usually one can feel an improvement in space-perception, deeper breathing, and more elasticity in one's tissue.

Now ask your partner to change the position and tap a different part of the body. Often the person being tapped tends to relax more and more and chooses positions closer and closer to the floor—which is all the more pleasant if there is an inviting mat awaiting—but I recommend doing some of the exercise while standing up, or on all fours. The person who is tapping should vary the areas he or she taps.

The back and shoulder areas are favorites, but I also recommend the head, the legs and the feet.

The tapper can use palms, finger tips or loose fists.

Make sure you stay in a dialogue with your partner so you can find the best strength to tap with.

# 7 Relaxed at your Desk, Without a Care on your Chair

T ime and again I meet people for whom an office job is out of the question because there is too much sitting involved. They prefer a physically active occupation; even half a day in front of the computer screen can be too much for them. Lack of movement is one of the most significant causes of a drop in happiness-inducing hormone levels. At the office, oxygen intake is just enough for the movement of the fingertips, while the rest of our muscles wonder what the point of their existence is. In the following chapter, we will familiarize ourselves with a series of exercises that transform the office desk and chair into gym apparatus for relaxation and fitness. We will also learn how to carry our after-work shopping bags more efficiently. These exercises will give the office worker more stamina—even those allergic to an office job will find that they can manage to remain relaxed and in a good mood.

## hand on the table

In the first exercise we will use the periphery (hand, arm) to stabilize ourselves as we move the middle section of the body (spine, thorax). This has a relieving effect on the locomotor system. In early childhood, we often originate our movements in the middle section of the body while being stabilized by the periphery. Adults gradually lose this way of moving: normally the periphery (shoulder girdle, arms) moves while the middle section (spine, pelvis, legs) remains stable.

These exercises refresh the nervous system while relaxing the shoulder girdle.

### wriggling zeppelin

We begin by moving the right arm a little, in order to see how our shoulder feels at the moment. This is a movement in which the middle section of the body remains still while the periphery moves. Next we do the opposite: we place a hand on a stable chair or low table, and move the body around the hand; the hand stays where it is while the trunk moves about. We can imagine that our lungs are a zeppelin: our arm is the anchor rope, our hand the anchor. A light wind is blowing, causing the zeppelin to move around onits rope. Thus we can move our trunk towards and away from our hand, or around the anchor rope.

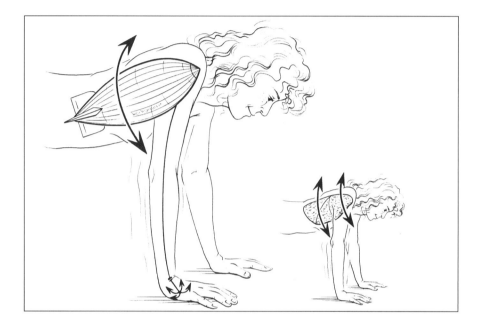

Be free and playful with your movements, without contorting your body in any painful way. After a few minutes, compare the flexibility of the right shoulder with the left by moving your now upraised arm around in the air. Finally, the exercise is repeated with the other arm.

## the right distance between hand and shoulder girdle (adapted from Bonnie Cohen)

Place both hands on a stable chair (or on the edge of a desk). By moving our trunk towards the chair, we reduce the gap between our shoulders and the chair. The distance between our hands and shoulder girdle has now shrunk. Maintaining this shoulder position, we stand up straight. Notice how the shoulders are now hunched.

Next we do the opposite: with outstretched arms, we place our hands on the chair, so that the distance between our hands and shoulders is as great as possible. Maintaining this shoulder position, we stand up straight, and we can see that the shoulders are now lower and more relaxed.

So, during your daily routine, remember once in a while to place your hands on a chair or desk, and then increase the distance between hands and shoulders.

# active pelvic floor – relaxed shoulders

In the following exercise we will see that an active pelvic floor helps the shoulders to relax. By placing a soft ball or a rolled-up towel under our bottom (under the tuberosity of the ischium), the pelvic floor is brought into action and its tone (tonus) is increased. This releases stress from the "upper floors" (back, shoulders, neck, head)—a lowering of the tonus. Your shoulders will say to themselves, "If you strengthen the foundations, I can safely relax!"

## the ball beneath the tuberosity of the ischium

Sit on a chair and place a ball under your right tuberosity. The ball should not be too hard, so that the tuberosity sinks a little into it. In order to keep the pelvis horizontal, the left tuberosity, which is not being supported by the ball, has now to be held a few centimeters (one or two inches) above the surface of the chair. In other words, the pelvic floor now has work to do. Next try moving the right tuberosity around on the ball. Then move the left tuberosity, imagining it to be a big crayon with which you can draw circles and loops—you could even write your name in the air. During these exercises, try to breathe in as relaxed a manner as possible. If you feel any discomfort in your lower back, increase the activity of the pelvic floor muscles or take a rest break.

Let the left tuberosity drop back down to the chair. Now the pelvis is in a crooked position. Then lift it up from the chair again. Now try to push apart the two tuberosities, and then to squeeze them together again. You feel the pelvic floor stretching and contracting. Next, remove the ball, and compare your shoulders. You can see that the shoulder on the side where the ball was is now lower. Perhaps you can even feel that the jaw and the whole right side of the face are more relaxed.

Now repeat the exercise on the left side. When you have done this, you take two balls and place them under both tuberosities. Now you can start moving around on the two balls in any way you want—like a fidgety schoolchild. After a few minutes, remove the balls. Both shoulders are relaxed and you find it easy to sit up straight.

# bringing space to the armpits

The armpit has the form of a pyramid whose peak points towards the shoulder joint. Its boundaries are described by the pectoralis major in front, the latissimus dorsi behind, the serratus anterior on the inside, and the brachial muscle on the outside. It is therefore an ideal point from which to send several muscles simultaneously to the land of relaxation.

### deep armpits (adapted from André Bernard)

Imagine the armpits becoming deep and supple. The "peak of the pyramid" is directly beneath the head of the humerus. We can feel the weight of the head and let it sink down. In this position, the joint capsule, the connective tissue sheet covering the joint, is indeed quite limp, hanging down like a soft rag.

### balls in the armpits

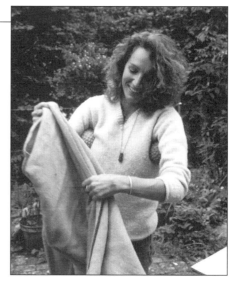

This exercise is especially practical if we cannot find time in our daily routine for relaxation exercises. The following exercise is active enough so we can keep going and suprises us with relaxed shoulders. Place two soft balls under the armpits. A small, rolled–up towel can also be used in place of a ball. Continue with your work, whether at the computer or around the house. It may be necessary to press the balls a little with the upper arms, so that they do not fall. If you feel any pain from the inner arms or ribcage, place the balls lower down, nearer the elbow. Work like that for about five minutes, then remove the balls. You will be surprised just how relaxed your shoulders now are. This exercise is based on the principle of reciprocal inhibition, where the activation of one muscle group causes the relaxation in the opposing muscle group.

## bringing space to the shoulders

Our hands are helpful allies in relieving tension in the shoulders; we need only allow them, with the active support of our imagination, to grasp things in a new way. Many potential tools for our relaxation exercises already exist in our mind; others are right in front of us, directly within our reach.

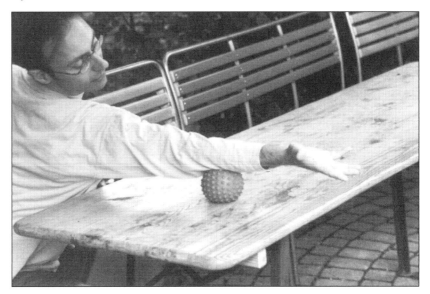

A bottle on a table can, for example, provide the perfect situation in which to relax the shoulders. The only condition is that the bottle is empty, so that it may be laid on its side. An excellent alternative to a bottle is a roll of paper towels, which also has the advantage of being somewhat softer. This relaxing exercise can be done before or during lunch, aiding in digestion. If you do not have a bottle or a towel roll, the exercise can be tried with a rolling pin, a ball (see photo) or even a roll of toilet paper—a sure way to elicit some laughs, which will improve the effect of the exercise

### rolling the bottle

Ensure that there are no other objects on the table, lay the bottle down and then place your forearm on the side of the bottle. Roll the bottle back and forth. Your shoulder, including the shoulder blade and collarbone, is part of this movement. I suggest that you inhale as you roll the bottle away, and exhale as you roll it back towards yourself. Now turn the arm, palm upward, and then roll the bottle back and forth. Then repeat the movement with the palm turned downward. Make the same movement with fingers stretched, then with the hand bunched in a fist. It is possible, for those who wish and who are flexible enough, that the rolling movement include the whole arm, right up to the armpit. In any case, it is important to breathe freely throughout the exercise; a wholehearted yawn would be very welcome!

Before continuing the exercise with the other arm, feel what effect the movement has had on your shoulder, and compare both sides.

### holding the kitten

Place your left hand on the right shoulder, covering the trapezius with cupped palm. The warmth of your hand helps the muscle to relax. Now take firmer hold of the muscle, as if kneading it once in slow motion. Keep a firm hold of the muscle for a few seconds. This movement is reminiscent of a mother cat holding her kitten by the scruff of the neck. The tissue in the kitten's neck is very elastic and strong, as if made for this particular purpose. Imagine that the tissue beneath your shoulder is just as flexible and soft as that in the kitten's neck. Then, very slowly, let go. This should produce a feeling of sliding and seeping. Repeat the holding and letting go action three or four times and you will feel a marked difference between the shoulders. A magnificent exercise for break time or even while travelling in a bus, train, or plane. Do it while you read your e-mail and you will have less strain on your eyes due to better posture. Neck, shoulder, and eye tension are closely related.

## standing and sitting

Our shoulders can only be as relaxed as our posture allows. Learning to stand and sit in a physically correct manner is one of the best ways to improve our posture, as these movements allow us to concentrate on the proper way of shifting our body weight. Children with a normal level of physical development retain a good posture when they write or draw. The spine is upright and the head inclined, without putting pressure on the neck. The shoulders hang by the side, relaxed. If school lessons are not regularly interrupted by breaks where the children can move around, they, too, will develop a bad posture in time. A lack of movement leads to tiredness and a passive approach to your work.

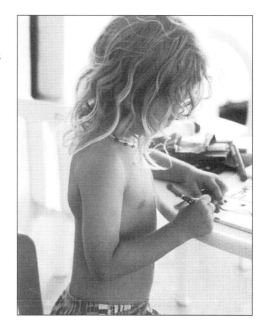

When we sit in an upright position, the weight of the upper body is put on the tuberosities of the ischium, the sitz-bones; when we stand, it is on the femoral heads, the top of the leg bone. The act of standing up therefore requires us to transfer our weight from the sitz-bones to the femoral heads. This is no easy task, as the tuberosities are lower down in the pelvis than the hip joints. Through specific exercise of the movement we make when we go from a sitting to a standing position, the muscles of the pelvis can be trained in such a way that the transfer of weight from legs to pelvis becomes better coordinated. This creates a better base for the spine, allowing it to become longer and more upright and strengthens the deep muscles of the pelvis. This, in turn, allows the the shoulders and neck to relax.

## rocking the sitz-bones

For this exercise we need a wooden chair. Its hard, flat seat means that we can easily feel our sitz-bones, inducing an active way of sitting. An overly comfortable chair, on the other hand, is an invitation to slouch.

We begin by rocking back and forward on our sitz-bones. At the same time, we place the fingers of our right hand on the right sacroiliac articulation and imagine that we are focusing fluid energy into this joint. We can easily feel it because of the adjacent bony bump of the posterior superior iliac spine, back on the pelvis. After a minute or so, we stop rocking, and see if the right shoulder has become more relaxed. Then we start rocking again, and place the fingers of our left hand on the left sacroiliac articulation. Again, we imagine that we are providing soft and fluid energy.

### melting the tuberosities (adapted from André Bernard)

We place our awareness on our left tuberosity, and feel its weight. We visualize its shape: the way it faces diagonally outwards, and is much thicker at the back than in front. Now we transfer our weight to the right tuberosity, so that the left is slightly raised from the chair. Next we imagine that this left sitz-bone is melting, dripping like beeswax. The more it melts, the more the left shoulder drops down with it.

We change sides and let the right sitz-bone hang – like the pendulum in a cuckoo clock. We shift our weight several times from the left to the right tuberosity, each time feeling how the raised sitz-bone hangs down.

### folding the hip

Now imagine that you have a thread attached to your left knee. At the precise moment that you transfer your weight to the right sitz-bone, raise the left knee up in the air—all the work being done by this imaginary thread. This creates a deep fold in the left hip: imagine a rag doll whose elbows and knees are made of deeply creased folds. At the same time, imagine that the left armpit is soft and spacious.

Now repeat the movement on the other side, raising the right knee as you transfer your weight to the left sitz-bone.

Repeat the action three times, shifting from the left to the right and back again.

Take a break from the leg movements and bend forward so that the head hangs down and the upper body rests on the legs. Imagine again how easily your hips can fold.

Stay in this position for a minute or two, and then come up very slowly. Feel the contact between the soles of your feet and the floor, and press the tuberosity down on the chair. These starting movements are enough for you to slowly become, vertebra by vertebra, upright. The spinous processes hang down in a relaxed way, and the coccyx feels as if it is grows through the chair to the floor.

Now repeat the first sequence of shifting weight onto the sitz-bone and lifting and folding the hip on the other side.

### from sitting to standing

Slide forward on the sitz-bones to the edge of the chair, and prepare yourself to move into a standing position by touching the hip joints, found in the middle of the groin. Visualize both the heads of the hip joint, to which you will soon transfer your weight. The trick is to use a

minimum amount of energy to stand up, taking advantage of
innate reflexes rather than heaving yourself up by straining
You are going to transfer your body weight forward to the legs with a
feeling of letting go. If you can manage this, your legs will at first bend a
little, and then the reflexes will adjust efficiently to this momentum and
automatically raise your body weight. This may seem a little awkward at
first, but it is worth trying.

Okay, get ready: your arms and shoulders are as relaxed as possible, and
you will try to stand up with the help of your legs and pelvis rather than
by tensing the upper body. Let your weight shift to the femoral heads and
feel the righting reflex in the legs, which effectively moves you into the
standing position.

As you sit down again, your arms hanging relaxed at your sides, use the
sitz-bones like tiny landing gear, locating the surface of the chair. Now sit
and stand several times, each time trying to transfer your weight more
efficiently from the sitz-bones to the top of the legs. At the same time, let
each arm hang like a pendulum, pointing to the center of the earth.

After several attempts, you will see how easy it is to sit on a chair with
totally relaxed arms hanging at your sides.

Finally, stand up while imagining the following: a thread is attached to
the pubic bone, at the front of the pelvis. Allow this thread, which points
diagonally upwards, to bring you into a standing position. Let the arms
hang and exhale through the armpits.

## shopping bags for posture exercises

In the following exercises we learn to unload the shoulders and neck
during shopping. The key to this is to activate the correct areas of the
body: pelvis, spine axis, legs and feet.

## giving weight to the ground

When lifting something it is vital not to carry the weight by tensing the neck and shoulder muscles. When we are about to lift a shopping bag, for instance, we should imagine that the weight is immediately transferred through our body to the feet—imagine that our feet carry the weight. We can support this image by pushing the feet into the ground while lifting the bag.

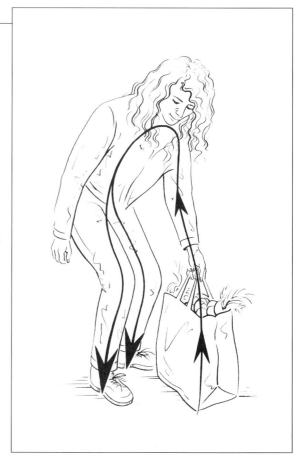

## arms hanging from the axis of the body

Ideally, we are carrying heavy bags distributed equally to both our hands in order not to create an unnecessary shifting of the spine. A well–aligned spine can carry a lot of weight; a crooked posture on the contrary is poison for our spine and intervertebral disks.

This becomes more relevant the heavier the load is. We can't balance our shopping on our head, as they do in Africa. Instead we are trying to use the spine in the right way by feeling, while carrying, that both arms are hanging equally from the axis of our body. The heavier the load is, the longer we visualize the axis. The main representative of this axis is, of course, our spine, which we imagine, while carrying, to be stretched both upwards and downwards.

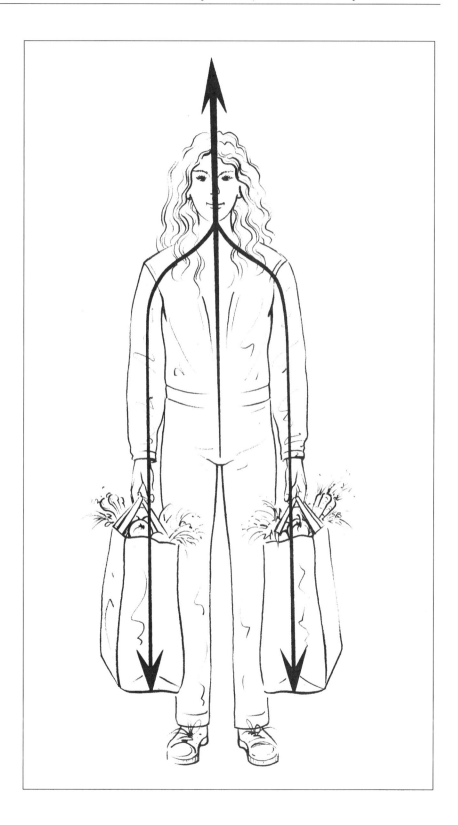

# 8  Help for the Neck

**N**eck pain is a common grievance. Aside from local pain, it can be responsible for nausea, migraine, and headaches. Most neck pain can be alleviated with the help of posture schooling, improved flexibility and elasticity, and also through becoming aware of relevant psychological factors. Fear, mental inflexibility, stubbornness, anger, and discontent reside in the neck.

These psychological problems can be solved through bodywork. As our neck becomes more supple, fear often disappears.

The biomechanical aspects of this area are important. Whoever holds their five kilogram (11 pound) head too far forward has condemned their neck muscles to a labor camp. As long as the neck muscles are tense, the weight of the head cannot be appropriately transferred to the spine. When the neck muscles become relaxed, a spontaneous feeling of uprightness arises in the thoracic spine.

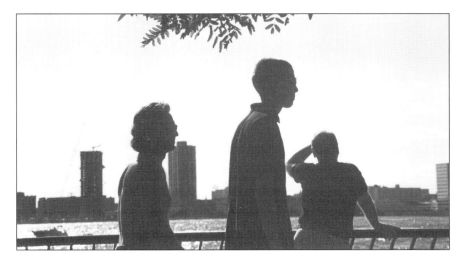

## neck freedom

How are you right now? Is your head able to sit lightly on the cervical spine even though you are reading—or are you plagued by neck pains that you would like to alleviate? And would you like to discover their root?

Before going into details concerning the problem of neck tension, I recommend the following exercise to give your neck a good dose of relaxation.

## energy stream in the neck

Before starting, move your neck around a bit and check out how your neck muscles feel. As already described in the section A Ball of Energy in the Hand (see page 6), rub the hands for a while until some warmth is created. Now hold them a few centimeters (1 to 2 inches) apart from each other and imagine that energy is flowing from one hand to the other, from left to right or from right to left as feels right. Try to activate this energy flow in a relaxed manner and let it flow constantly in one direction without any effort. Relaxed breathing helps to do this.

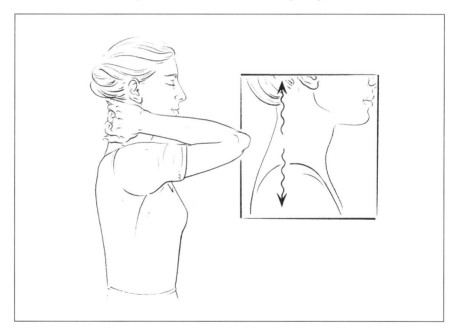

Now lift the hands and put them on both sides of the neck. The fingers will overlap a bit. Keep picturing the stream of energy, but now it is flowing through the neck muscles like a soft breeze. Stay in this position for at least a minute and rock the head gently. After taking away your hands, nod lightly and see if the neck muscles now feel relaxed.

### skull base and brain

The brain has some freedom of movement in the skull. It is important that we don't lose this flexibility and that we train it with the help of visualization.

Put your hands on the back of your head and lift it a bit while visualizing the brain gliding in the opposite direction. It is as if a ball is moving inside our skull. Now lower the back of the head a bit and visualize the opposite movement: the brain moving upwards. Repeat these movements about five times before taking your hands away. Now see how your neck feels.

### relaxing the neck

Sometimes there are unusual opportunities to rest the neck—as I once experienced at a highway rest stop: a warm stone literally invited me to relax my neck on it. Stay on the lookout for opportunities to relax your neck. There are no limits to the possibilities.

## the neck starts in the back

Many neck problems have their origin in the upper cervical spine, because the lordosis (forward curve) of the neck depends on the situation in the thoracic spine below, and also because many muscles extend from upper back to the neck. Even though in the next exercise you will probably feel a certain amount of tension in the thorax area and will at first not feel very comfortable, try to relax and to breathe calmly. This situation is a metaphor for life: staying calm in an uncomfortable situation.

In both the following experiments we will experience, through the shortening of a muscle, a stretching and relaxation. This is possible because the muscles react to spontaneous—not chronic—shortening with elongation.

### the ball between the shoulder blades

Put a very soft ball—or, if not available, a rolled up towel—between your shoulder blades. Stay very calm and try to enjoy the situation. To heighten the effect, move the arms around a bit. Lift them and stretch them upward by the side of the head. After three minutes, take the ball away and observe the change in the shoulders.

### soft ball, soft neck

Now put the soft ball or rolled towel under the neck. The neck should be able to rest on it without the chin being pushed upwards. (If this exercise causes any pain, don't do it.) Imagine the cervical spine slowly sinking into the ball.

After three minutes take the ball away and enjoy the effect.

# four joints

When looking at the skull from below, one can see four large joint surfaces. On the edge of the hole in the skull can be found the two condyles of the skull base. These two tuberosities fit exactly into the hollows of the top vertebra, the atlas, and make nodding movements possible. In this position the head can be tipped backwards to a considerable degree without the cervical spine needing to extend—a movement which can often be observed in small children. For adults, though, this movement is difficult because of our poor head posture, but if done properly it can be a welcome change for the neck muscles.

I call the condyles of the skull base the "sitting tuberosities" of the head. The two other joints are the mandibular joint sockets; contrary to the condyles of the skull they are hollows into which the condyles of the jaw fit. These four joints are crucial to our head posture and the state of our neck. It is essential to discover and get a feel for them.

The top vertebra, the atlas, has one long transverse process, but only a slight spinous process. It doesn't have a vertebral body and looks like a ring with wings. Considering that it carries the head, it is a very delicate bone. The joint between the atlas and the base of the skull is one of the most flexible points of the spine—because it is essential that the spinal chord not be jammed. A bad posture can become established here very quickly for the same reason. The second top vertebra, the axis, on the contrary has a long spinous process, which can be felt easily, and hardly any transverse processes.

The dens is a toothlike process that sticks up from the axis bone and protrudes into the atlas and builds an axis of rotation (that's where the name comes from) for the atlas. The two transverse processes of the atlas and the spinous process of the axis are important pointers to the state of the neck. You can feel the transverse processes of the atlas under the mastoid of the temporal bone. The spinous process of the axis stands out as a prominent spot in the upper part of the neck.

## sliding down the neck

Let your fingers slide down the back of the head until you find a small hollow. In this hollow, under the skin, is a bony protuberance: this is the spinous process of the axis. Touch the hollow very gently and imagine that you are breathing in and out of the hollow. Breathe through the spinous process of the axis as if it was the mouthpiece of a flute.

Then, touch the mastoid of the temporal bone, found behind the ear lobe. Just under the mastoid you can feel the transverse processes of the atlas. The joint that connects the skull with the atlas can be found just between your fingers. Imagine that there is an air cushion carrying the skull so that the joint is relieved of its burden. You can actually hear the joint sighing with relief as weight is lifted off of it. A participant in one of my workshops, Judith Conrad, once suggested a brilliant image for the condyles of the skull: the round and slippery part of a deodorant stick which fits exactly into the hollows of the atlas and allows playful gliding movements. Nod with your head minimally forward and backward and feel how the deodorant stick glides. Of course, imagine your favorite scent with the image! This exercise is a good example of combining visual with heard, smelled and felt imagery, enhancing its overall effect.

## the muscles of the atlas and the axis

Behind the condyles of the skull are short, deep neck muscles that are responsible for the fine tuning of the head posture. They are called the muscles of the occipital bone, which come in pairs. The occipital bone will be referred to as "OB."

The big OB muscle originates at the spinous process of the axis and continues to the OB. The small muscle starts at the spinous process of the atlas and then connects to the OB. Both can bend the head backwards, sideways, and turn it a little. The lower oblique muscle goes from the spinous process of the axis to the transverse process of the atlas. The upper oblique muscle goes from the transverse process of the atlas to the OB. These muscles are often chronically tense because they hardly ever get stretched in everyday life. If we bend the head forward from the neck,these muscles are stretched. But most adults bend the cervical spine and indeed the whole back to look down— keeping the upper neck short. In complete contrast to this, an infant will look down with the help of the skull joint and atlas vertebra, and so stretches the muscles.

The OB muscles are in such close proximity to the skull opening and the spinal chord that tension in this area is a serious disturbance for the nervous system, because very little pressure is needed to hamper

the conductivity of a nerve.
Not only can neck and
back pain be the result, but
also headaches, migraines,
and a general lack of
energy.

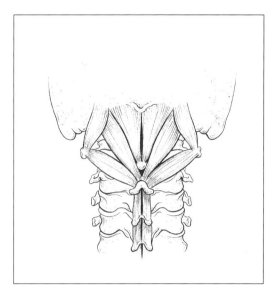

## gliding with the neck muscles

This exercise can relax the entire spine.

Slide your fingers from the back of the head down until you come to the neck muscles. Bend the head back a bit, keeping a relaxed jaw, so that you can dive a little bit deeper into the neck muscles with your fingers. If this is very painful, keep your fingers light. Now make small circular movements and imagine these muscles becoming very soft. Breathe very gently and let the jaw hang.

Now rock the head gently on the atlas and feel how the neck muscles get shorter and longer. Remember the sliding feeling in the muscle (see page 43), and try to feel it in the neck muscles. It could be that your neck doesn't feel very slippery—this is normal at first. Don't give up! Give it another try!

Now something for the more advanced visualizers (of course, everyone can try this). The sliding agent for muscles is called ATP (adenosine triphosphate). It makes the separation of single muscle filaments possible. ATP is produced by small cell organelles called mitochondria. ATP is literally the "muscle softener" molecule.

Imagine that plenty of ATP is flowing into your neck muscle fibers. This lubricant makes muscle sliding possible. As long as there is ATP, there will be movement in the muscles.

### the star

Who would have thought that there is a star shining at the back of the neck?! This star consists of several muscles which all radiate from the spinous process of the axis vertebra. Imagine a really bright star, or with the help of breathing create a feeling of expansion around the atlas. It helps to imagine the atlas becoming broader, as if it was being pulled apart by the transverse processes like chewing gum. You can feel a flow originating from the hollow of the neck, which supports the back of the head. At the same time the spinous processes sink down.

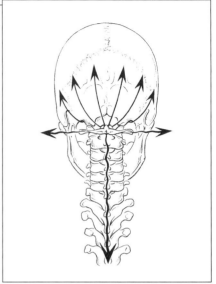

For those hungry for knowledge, the muscles on the illustration on the previous page are the following: attaching to the transverse process of the first cervical vertebra and creating a box–like shape are the obliquus capitis inferior and superior. The muscle that runs obliquely upward from the spinous process of the second cervical vertebra to the base of the skull is the rectus capitis major. In between this muscle you can see the rectus capitis minor which connects the spinous process of the first cervical vertebra with the base of the skull.

## the sternomastoid muscle

The sternomastoid is a large muscle that can usually be found easily. When you turn your head to the left, you can feel a thick bulge that starts at the breastbone and continues to the mastoid process. This is the sternomastoid muscle. It is the muscle which thrusts the head forwards when we make an aggressive face.

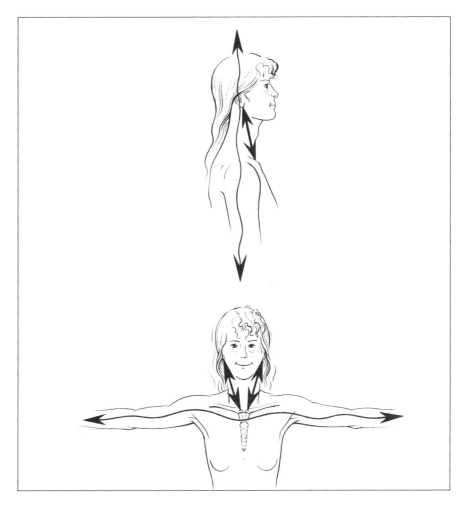

At the same time it can turn and bend the head to the side. It has two points of origin: one at the collarbone and one at the breastbone. The two "heads" of the muscle unite and end at the mastoid of the temporal bone. It is important from time to time to let this muscle feel its full length. When it does, astonishing feelings of expansion can occur in the neck and arm, the head seems to find its true place on top of the spine, and the arms have increased freedom of movement.

## elongation of the sternomastoid

The cervical spine is supposed to stay upright and not bend during the following elongation of the sternomastoid.

First bend your head a bit forwards so that the chin comes closer to the thorax. This movement should take place exclusively in the joint of the skull base and atlas. Then bend the head a bit to the left, so that a long curve appears in the cervical spine. Then turn the head to the right and look back in the direction just moved from. Breathe gently and feel how the right sternomastoid is stretched—like cotton wool that is being pulled apart.

A mistake that is often made in this exercise is that the head loses its forward bend during turning. It's not an easy movement, but it is important to keep an eye on the proper execution of the exercise.

Now repeat the sequence on the other side: move your head forward so that the jaw comes close to the thorax. This movement should be made from the joint of the skull base and the atlas. Then bend the head a bit to the right, so that a long curve appears in the cervical spine. Then turn the head to the left and look back in the direction just moved from. Breathe gently and feel how the left sternomastoid is stretched.

## loosening the jaw muscles

The jaw is a veritable sponge for soaking up all sorts of tension.

We often keep our mouth shut when we actually want to say something, and we tense the jaw when we eat while supposedly dieting. When we feel anger or sorrow, we clench the jaw—but also when speaking, if we have a bad posture. The jaw joint is used more often than any other in the body. Mabel Todd pointed out that the heaviest part of the jaw is at the back of the lower jawbone—one can imagine it hangs from the temporal bone.

The strongest muscles in the body—apart of the uterus muscles—are the jaw closers. The jaw openers, on the other hand, are very weak. The opening of the jaw is achieved chiefly through the relaxation of the jaw closers. Apparently, once upon a time clenching the teeth was more important than yawning. Many people experience the beginnings of a migraine or headache as tension in the jaw.

When these muscles are loosened it does miracles for the neck and shoulders. But be careful! It is similar to dusting a room: when one starts to clean a dusty room, a lot of dust is stirred up at first. Relaxation of the jaw joint can lead to yawning, tiredness and even dizziness at first. But overcoming this phase certainly has its rewards.

In the following experiment it is important to know that you can take a break at any time—don't exhaust yourself by touching the jaw joint and muscles for a long time.

## opening the ears

Put a finger into your ear hole and press your finger gently forward. Open the jaw and you can feel movement and that the ear hole gets bigger. The reason for this is that the jaw joint is just in front of the ear. While moving your jaw feel how the jaw joint moves at the front of the edge of the ear cartilage. The jaw moves forwards while opening. The condyle moves down and forwards when we open the mouth wide. We can also feel the ear hole becoming wider and spacious when opening the jaw slowly. This is so that we can hear better when we open the mouth! When we let the jaw drop from astonishment, we're getting ready to hear more unbelievable news.

Again put a finger into the ear and say loudly: "Yeah, yeah, yeah, yeah," as if you were a bit bored, with a limp feeling in the jaw. You should be able to feel how the condyle slides back and forth in front of the ear hole.

## massaging the edge of the jaw

Put your hand in the "Oh dear!" position on the right cheek, thumb resting on the curve of the jawbone. This corner of the jaw can be felt easily. Massage this spot for a bit and then slide your thumb along the inner edge of the jaw to the front as if you were kneading the edge of the dough for a fruit cake—pressing inwards from time to time. At first you will feel a spongy tissue; this is a salivary gland which lies under the tongue. Along the whole edge of the bone to the tip of the jaw is a muscle that constitutes, like a hammock, the floor of the jaw (the mylohyoid).

With our touch we can balance the tone of this muscle.

Kneed the right side of the jaw two or three times from the curve of the jaw to the tip and back again. Let both arms hang by your side and you will feel to your amazement that your right side is more relaxed. The muscle on the floor of the mouth helps to relax the neck and jaw.

Repeat the exercise on the left side.

### melting the masseter

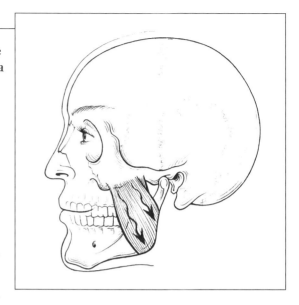

First touch the cheekbone with your hands. This is a relatively small facial bone, which constitutes the outside of the eye socket. The cheekbone forms, together with the temporal bone, a bow towards the ear.

Put your fingers on the bone under the eye and slide along this track of bone backwards until you are about one centimeter (half an inch) in front of the ear. Your hand is now on the part of the bow that is made up by the temporal bone.

Leave the cheekbone and stroke the cheek downward and a little backward towards the curve of the jaw: this is the course of a very strong muscle, the masseter.

Repeat this stroking movement three or four times and let the jaw hang loose. Imagine that your fingers are sliding through a piece of butter. If you find an obstinate spot in the masseter, then stay there with the fingertips for a moment and imagine that this area of tension is melting.

Do these stroking movements on both sides of the face at the same time.

### the posture of the jaw influences the posture of the whole body

Now we will focus on a small muscle, but an important one, for the posture of the jaw. About a centimeter (half an inch) in front of the ear, below the cheekbone is a hollow. In the depth of this hollow lies a muscle that plays an important part in the grinding movements of the jaw. It is called the lateral pterygoid.

If we can manage to relax this muscle, it has an almost magical effect on the shoulders and neck. The lateral pterygoid, "ptery" for short, is a muscle that pulls the jaw towards the front.

Push your lower jaw a bit forwards and observe the feeling that accompanies this movement. It is a facial expression used in aggressive behavior, so it is not surprising that this muscle tends to get charged with unpleasant tensions. The ptery is a very key muscle for tension in the jaw and throughout the entire body.

## loosening the ptery

Move your jaw sideways to the left and to the right. Is it equally easy to move it in both directions?

If you put your finger just in front of the ear hole, your finger is on the condyle of the lower jaw. Open the jaw a little and you will discover the small hollow of the ptery. If you open the jaw completely, then this hollow gets covered by the head of the mandible. Open the jaw halfway so that you can put a fingertip into the hollow.

Imagine now that this hollow becomes deep and soft. Breathe through this hollow and see how all your tension goes sailing out of it—your fingers are like small lasers finding the tension and melting it.

Put your hands behind the skull to support it and bend the head backwards. Try to let the jaw drop without opening it too far. This stretches the ptery. In this position, push the jaw slightly forward and let it fall back again slowly. The hands at the back of the neck push the skull into an upright position.

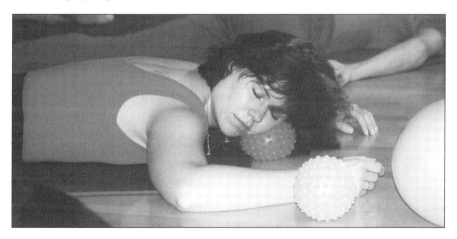

Another way to loosen the masseter and the ptery is to lie the jaw on a ball and slowly move the jaw. I recommend you start with a very soft ball.

## letting the temporalis flow

The temporalis is a jaw closer with a broad origin on the skull—in front of and above the ear. One can see it protruding near the temple when chewing. It goes under the cheekbone and attaches itself to one of the processes of the jaw (the coronoid process). Massage with your fingers circularly above the ears, in line with the eyes, a few times.

Imagine how this muscle flows under the cheekbone and how the cheekbone floats upwards. Repeat this stroking a few times.

Put your fingers on your soft cheek and slide backwards until you come against the joint process of the jaw, on to which the temporalis is attached. This is felt best, right under the cheekbone, when the jaw is slightly open. Massage this spot—and don't be surprised if it is a bit painful. If you hit the right spot it will cause an instant sense of relaxation in the jaw and neck.

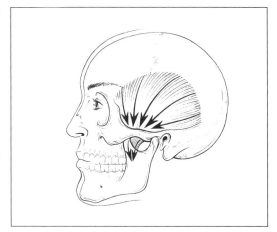

## neck balloon

Imagine there is a tiny balloon floating under the back of your head, which is holding the back of the head up. At the same time let the jaw hang down. The spine stretches, the breathing becomes calm. Make sure that you are not exerting yourself by holding the neck up, and leave the strength of the support to your imagination.

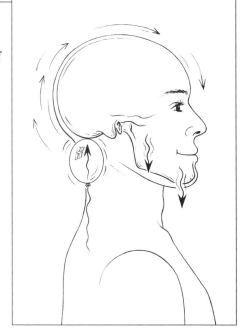

## relaxing the tongue

We often tense the tongue without noticing it. The tongue is connected via different muscles and ligaments with the base of the skull and the jaw, which is why it influences the state of tension in the neck and shoulders. The tongue is attached to the hyoid bone on top of the larynx—a muscle that is connected at only one end to a bone. When swallowing, we create an artificial joint between the palate and the tongue.

You can feel this connection if you try to swallow with an open mouth without touching the palate with the tongue.

What movements can we make with the tongue? We can stretch it out of the mouth and pull it back again. We can move it sideways, up and down. These movements are mainly done with the outer lingual muscles, those muscles that connect to the tongue from outisde. The tongue can change into almost any shape since it is packed with muscles right to the tip. The inner muscles of the tongue lie in different layers. The tongue becomes flat when the vertical muscles are shortened. If I want to make a thick tongue I have to shorten the muscles which run transversely from front to back.

### nodding and the tongue

Nod your head with a relaxed neck and a relaxed tongue. Then nod with a tense tongue—clump the tongue tightly in your mouth. You can feel how the neck also gets tense. Then press the tongue into the right cheek, turn the head to the right and then to the left. Which side is it easier to turn to? You can feel how the position of the tongue has an influence on the movement of the neck.This influence on the neck is also based on the fact that the tissue of the tongue was created embryonically out of a segment of the back of the head.

The human body is like a worm built up in segments. Luckily that isn't so obvious any more. The tongue was created out of the same segment as the occipital bone and the muscles that are attached to it.The nerve that innervates the tongue (twelfth cranial nerve, nervus hypoglossus), also radiates downwards; so the "wiring" was extended downwards, in a manner of speaking. When we put our fingers on the occipital bone and the neck muscles, this path can be traced. From here the tongue originated and grew in two parts around the spine to the front—around the gut to where it can now be found. So the tongue is related more closely to the back of the head than the neck.

### soft tongue, soft neck

Put your middle fingers into the hollow of the neck and your thumbs under the jaw on to the muscle of the floor of the mouth. Imagine that the tongue is very relaxed and soft and become aware of the soft oral floor. Try to rock the head lightly without losing this feeling of softness. You can even imagine that the tongue is hanging from the neck. When you move the tongue around a bit, perhaps you can feel a reaction in your neck, especially when pulling the tongue back too far.

### the tongue in the hammock

The tongue sits on the hyoid bone, which in turn is attached by muscles and ligaments to the jaw and the back of the head. That is why the tongue seems to rest in a bony rocking chair. Touch the hyoid bone just above the larynx and imagine how the tongue sits on this bone. Move your head in different directions and note the reactions of the tongue. Can you keep the tongue relaxed, or do the movements of the head create some tension in the tongue? Focus on the root of the tongue—above the larynx—and stay relaxed.

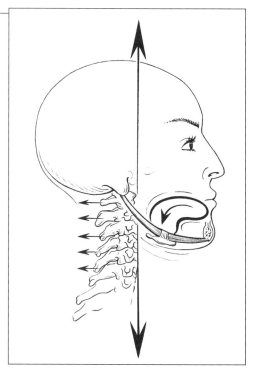

# 9  Giving oneself up to play

**T**he best medicine is surrender. If one watches children playing "catch," or who are dancing, singing, shrieking, one sees limitless energy and spontaneous joy—complete abandon. Where does all this energy, this whirling looseness, this ceaseless, curious exploring come from? Is it freedom and having no responsibility? Is it a genetic program that is turned off as we get older? What is happening? Our lives become more and more settled, time reigns supreme—many people are only working in jobs to earn money— "catch" games have little financial reward! This is why the following experiment is dedicated to spontaneous devotion to daily activity.

## devotion in daily life

Is there anything you would really like to do right now? Nothing? The thing you would really like to do right now isn't possible? Never mind. I suggest the following: find any activity that you can do right now, even something you would have had to do anyway—like watering the flowers, taking out the garbage, or something as trivial as moving a chair to a new spot in the room—and do it with total devotion, full of joy and lust for life. The cycle of devotion and spontaneity is the via regia to relaxation.

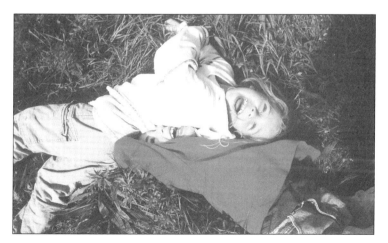

## other books by Eric Franklin

*Dance Imagery for Technique and Performance*
Human Kinetics
Champaign, IL, USA

*Dynamic Alignment through Imagery*
Human Kinetics
Champaign, IL, USA

## workshops

Workshops and teacher trainings, open to everybody, are regularly offered on the topics covered in this book as well as other aspects of movement and therapy.

Visit our web page at:
WWW.franklin-methode.ch

Or contact us at:
Institut für Franklin-Methode
Brunnenstrassse 1
CH–8610 Uster
Switzerland

email: info@franklin-methode.ch

The exercise balls and bands mentioned in the book can be obtained at the address above or to order in the US,
e-mail: pinhasiamos@hotmail.com

# Index